Praise for *More Health, Less Care*

We all need help to reach our health goals, but individual responsibility is the key. Dr. Weiss has described a way for all of us to take responsibility for our own health while living and working in contemporary society. The Personal Prescription can work to get you healthier, keep you healthier and prepare you to deal more effectively with health issues that we all will face at some time in our lives.

THOMAS EBERT, MD
CHIEF MEDICAL OFFICER
HEALTH NEW ENGLAND, INC., SPRINGFIELD, MA

Peter Weiss provides an effective and motivating way to think about how everyone can play a much more direct role in their own health and wellness care. The lessons found in this book will make a positive difference in the life of anyone who reads it.

PATRICIA KOHN
CHIEF OPERATING OFFICER
MANAGED CARE AND HEALTH PLAN
GUNDERSEN LUTHERAN HEALTH SYSTEM, LA CROSSE, WI

Finally, a physician engages us in a real discussion about our responsibility for our own health and then provides a clear road map to help find our way.

ALLAN EINBODEN
CHIEF EXECUTIVE OFFICER
SCOTT & WHITE HEALTH PLAN, TEMPLE, TX

Dr. Weiss inspires us to take charge of our health and reap the benefits of our life-changing efforts. Experience the powerful effects of managing your own healthcare!

TONY FERRETTI, PhD, CLINICAL PSYCHOLOGIST

Written with clarity and insight, Peter Weiss' message is that good health depends on making simple and practical changes in our lives. By following a down-to-earth, practical approach to staying healthy, *More Health, Less Care* instills the courage and commitment needed to change bad habits that can impact one's lifelong health and wellness.

JAMES V. PALERMO, MD
EDITOR-IN-CHIEF
SPACE COAST MEDICINE & HEALTHY LIVING

While the politicians debate, here's all you need to start your own personal health care reform. In *More Health, Less Care*, Dr. Peter Weiss shares an insider's view of the limits of modern medicine and helps you move closer towards total health in body, mind and spirit. No silver bullets, but complete, concise, 'start tonight' recommendations for achieving and maintaining maximal personal health.

ROSEMARY D. LAIRD, MD, MHSA
MEDICAL DIRECTOR
HEALTH FIRST AGING INSTITUTE

More Health, Less Care

More Health, Less Care

HOW TO TAKE CHARGE OF
YOUR MEDICAL CARE
AND WRITE YOUR OWN
PERSONAL PRESCRIPTION
FOR LIFELONG HEALTH

Peter J. Weiss, MD, FACP

LACHANCE PUBLISHING • NEW YORK
www.lachancepublishing.com

Library of Congress Control Number: 2009939810

Published by LaChance Publishing LLC
120 Bond Street, Brooklyn, NY 11217
www.lachancepublishing.com

This book is available at special discounts for bulk purchases for sales promotions or premiums. Special editions, including personalized covers, excerpts of existing books, and corporate imprints, can be created in large quantities for special needs. For more information, write to LaChance Publishing or email at info@lachancepublishing.com.

Contents

Contents

Contents

Foreword

From a health standpoint, the typical American has gone rapidly downhill over the last 20 years. On average, we have grown fatter, developed higher blood sugar and cholesterol, and we are still smoking far too much. The bottom line is that we are destroying the benefits of three decades of advancements in healthcare with our ever-worsening lifestyles. How is it that America, while spending the most money per person on healthcare globally, ranks lower than over forty other countries in life expectancy and healthcare satisfaction? Dr. Peter J. Weiss gives us an answer in *More Health, Less Care*.

This short volume may well be one of the most valuable self-help books you will ever read. It's a groundbreaking work that ties together Dr. Weiss' experiences as a physician, as a healthcare executive and as a patient himself. In *More Health, Less Care*, Dr. Weiss demonstrates how traditional medical care often just "doesn't work right" for improving patients' health. Although both patient and doctor mean well, many individuals with "lifestyle illnesses" such as diabetes and cardiovascular disease get slowly and progressively worse. Fortunately, Dr. Weiss has a solution to this all-too-common situation. With clear writing and simple examples, he presents an effective and "doable" strategy for individuals to help themselves to better health and well-being.

If you don't have bad habits, high blood pressure or diabetes, and if you're fit and trim with healthy, 90 year-old parents, you can put this book down now. However, the rest of us need it. The insights and advice offered here can save your life. Take them seriously.

Joseph S. Alpert, MD
Professor of Medicine,
University of Arizona College of Medicine, Tucson, Arizona
Editor-in-Chief, *American Journal of Medicine*

Introduction

Why write this book?

I want to help you be healthy. For over 25 years, I have been trying to help people improve their health—first as a practicing
physician and subsequently as the Medical Director and Chief
Executive Officer of Health First Health Plans, a quality-driven
health insurance company. Many other physicians and healthcare leaders have been trying to do the same. But despite all this
effort, I have witnessed the explosion of obesity, diabetes, and
high blood pressure among Americans, even as I've seen the development of many new treatments for these conditions. And I
haven't seen very many people getting truly well and enjoying
excellent health. Obviously, something's wrong here. What
we're doing isn't working. Frankly, for many people "traditional
healthcare" for common chronic medical conditions doesn't
work. In fact, relying solely on traditional healthcare can be part
of the problem.

By "traditional healthcare" I mean the typical series of events that comprise care for most people with health concerns in our society. You have a health issue, identify it as a "medical problem" and see a doctor. The physician makes a diagnosis and prescribes medicines or treatments, expecting you to follow his instructions. Unfortunately, looking at all health concerns as "medical problems" to be solved by a doctor can be a problem in itself. In this book I show how and why traditional healthcare isn't working for many people, and I describe a personal approach to improving your health that does work. I call this method the "Personal Prescription." If you were my patient, this is what we would be talking about.

How is the "personal prescription" different from "traditional healthcare?"

In traditional healthcare, the individual is often defined as an object ("the patient") with a problem to be solved by the doctor, and as a result may not feel personally responsible for finding a solution to improving his or her health. But people are not mass-produced cars waiting to be fixed by mechanics. The car doesn't have to do anything to get repaired. As long as it's in the shop, the mechanics will fix it. People are different. Any solution, even if it's just taking a single pill, must be acted upon by "the patient" himself, and every patient is different. People don't come off an assembly line identical to each other, and neither do their health and medical concerns. Consequently, individuals *must* participate in designing and implementing the solution to their problems.

Too often, providers may identify or diagnose medical problems independent of the patient himself and without regard to other problems that particular individual may have. It seems that some providers assume that "diabetes is diabetes" and "high blood pressure is high blood pressure" regardless of the particular patient with these conditions. This can create a "one size fits all approach" to treating illness, which may be too little, too much or not quite the right treatment to address the unique needs of the individual patient.

This is compounded for the many patients who have multiple specialists, each of whom may treat just one small part of the individual's overall health. Often none of these specialists feel responsible for the whole person, and they typically don't communicate well with each other.

Lastly, root causes may go unaddressed by both the physician and the individual. Sure, the patient may need treatment for diabetes, but why does this patient have diabetes in the first place? Where did it come from? What could possibly be done to help eliminate the cause of the diabetes, thereby curing the patient of the condition?

Add it all up and you have a treatment plan that doesn't fit the unique needs of that particular patient and therefore won't be effective. The patient either doesn't understand it or won't be able to comply with it. And it doesn't cure the problem by addressing the root cause, anyway.

By contrast, in the Personal Prescription the individual learns to accept responsibility for his or her own health, and physicians become resources for the individual in solving his or her problem. The Personal Prescription emphasizes identifying the root cause of medical problems, using available resources to find an effective solution, and implementing the solution in an effective and lasting way. As a "whole person" approach without the one size fits all mentality, the Personal Prescription avoids the typical shortfalls of traditional medical care.

Like most worthwhile things, there are no shortcuts to attaining good health and well-being, but the Personal Prescription is simple and straightforward. With commitment and dedication, it will work for you.

How was the personal prescription developed? Are these original ideas?

The Personal Prescription is my original expression of what I have learned through my experiences as a medical doctor and an individual concerned with my own health. Of course, many other authors, teachers, patients, family and friends have contributed to my thinking over the years. Some of the authors, teachers and their works that have helped me are listed at the end of this book. Although I don't claim that any of the individual ideas are original, I think you will find the Personal Prescription to be a unique—and uniquely helpful—approach to improving your health.

What makes this book special?

This book is for you, but I've put a lot of myself into it. Although we will likely never meet in person, I care for you and hope to develop a relationship with you through this work. As in any good relationship, I've tried to be completely honest and open with you about becoming healthy.

Many other personal health books recommend a certain diet or particular exercise regimen, but no book has all the "answers" *for you*. This book is designed to help you learn how to find your own answers. Think of this book as the treasure map and your good health as the treasure.

Who is this book intended for?

This book is for everyone who wants to improve his or her health. I primarily address individuals with conditions that are caused or made worse by lifestyle choices—conditions such as type II diabetes,* high blood pressure, high cholesterol, heart disease, obesity, arthritis and others. I target these "lifestyle conditions" because they are the most common and significant problems that people face with their physical health.

---

*It's important to differentiate type I from type II diabetes. Type II diabetes typically occurs in adults from excessive weight gain and is often curable through lifestyle change. Type I diabetes usually develops in childhood due to insulin deficiency resulting from damage or destruction of the insulin producing cells of the pancreas. Type I diabetes is not a "lifestyle disease" and treatment with insulin is required for life.

What if I have a serious non-lifestyle illness like cancer? Can this book help me?

Yes it can. Those with serious illness must also be ultimately responsible or "in charge" of the care they receive. Just having all the usual traditional healthcare is not enough for the best results here either. The individual must understand and participate in his or her own care. Also, emotional and spiritual issues often rise in importance as physical illnesses become more serious, and these are often poorly addressed in traditional healthcare.

Can others benefit from this book?

Of course! Spouses, lovers and friends of those with lifestyle illnesses can be of better help to those they love after becoming familiar with the concepts discussed here.

Emotional and spiritual issues are very common in today's society. Emotional disorders such as depression and anxiety can have adverse effects on physical health. Individuals with these conditions can also benefit from this book.

This book can also be of value to doctors and other healthcare practitioners. Most physicians will recognize the necessity of the Personal Prescription in helping their patients to truly achieve lasting health and well-being. The concepts provide a helpful framework for doctors to use in their interactions with patients. Clinicians of all types should encourage their patients to read this book and help them implement the method to find solutions.

Even those who are not ill but seek to live a healthy and balanced lifestyle will find value here. And finally, the principles outlined in this book provide a general philosophy of problem-solving and self-improvement that can be applied to any condition, problem or situation in your life where you desire a positive change.

What is the purpose of this book?

The purpose of this book is to help you get and stay healthy—physically, emotionally and spiritually. If you are seeking improvement in any of these areas, this book is for you. In writing the book, I've mostly used examples related to physical health—improving diet, increasing exercise and losing weight—because these goals are so common in our country today. However, I believe that emotional and spiritual health are the building blocks of good physical health. The philosophy outlined in the book can also be used for improvement in these areas. I hope these pages help you along your life's journey.

The doctor of the future will give no medicine,
but will interest her or his patients in the care
of the human frame, in a proper diet,
and in the cause and prevention of disease.

Thomas A. Edison

Acknowledgments

Nothing great happens without help, so let me acknowledge those who've helped me with *More Health, Less Care*.

I'd like to first thank all who helped me learn the lessons I've shared here, starting with my wife, Sharon. Thank you, Sharon. I'm blessed to have you as my partner in life. Linda Cobb, Bill Davies, Bill Ranieri, my friends at Eastminster Presbyterian Church, and my former patients have also been very helpful in shaping my thinking. Although I've never met any of them, the individuals identified in the Resources section have profoundly helped me to live a better life.

Then there are those who helped in the actual writing and production of the finished work. Keith Lundquist, Jim Gillespie, Bill Ranieri, Gene Davis, Ann Pallex, Margaret Haney, Bill Anderson, Mike Edwards, Dr. Joe Collins, Lisa Slattery, Dr. John McKinney, Peter Straley, Dr. Larry Bishop, and Dr. Tom Ebert reviewed early drafts of the manuscript and provided major assistance. A number of others made less major but similarly helpful comments along the way. Members of the Space Coast Writers' Guild shared valuable insider tips on writing and publishing in addition to offering encouragement. Dr. Rosemary Laird introduced me to Victor Starsia of LaChance Publishing. I am indebted to Victor, editors Richard Day Gore and Juliann Garey, and the staff at LaChance for believing in this work and crafting the final version you are holding. Thank you all.

Of course, many people provided and continue to provide me with love and support. My wife, Sharon, and my children, Allison and Kevin, accepted without complaint the many hours when I was "writing the book again." My close colleagues and friends at Health First Health Plans, Mike Means, Joy Gilbert, Jim Gillespie, Angela Handa, Dr. Miguel Fernandez, Roberta Stoner and Paulette Varney, encouraged me as good teammates do. Many other friends, acquaintances and business associates listened to my dreams for this work and were uniformly supportive.

Finally, I thank God for everything.

More Health,
Less Care

CHAPTER ONE

The Shortfalls of Traditional Healthcare

Traditional healthcare often doesn't help people to become truly healthy. Many medical problems persist and even worsen despite all the usual traditional healthcare. Let's examine the case of Bob Baker, a typical patient within the "traditional healthcare system," which clearly illustrates the issues.

Bob's Untimely Demise

Bob Baker is a patient of Dr. Lisa Martin. Bob works as an engineer for a Fortune 500 company that holds major commercial and Department of Defense contracts. He's 45 years old and happily married with two college-age children. Bob's lifestyle is stressful. He travels for business frequently, is expected to entertain clients, and always does "whatever it takes" to keep the clients and his boss happy. Unfortunately, keeping others happy has resulted in Bob's diabetes, high blood pressure and his being 40 pounds above his ideal bodyweight of 170 pounds.

Bob was fit and trim when he married Susan twenty years ago, but his weight increased gradually over the last 15 years as he spent more time taking care of business and less time taking care of himself. The diabetes and the high blood pressure developed as a result of the weight gain. Susan has been very concerned about his health for years and it's been a contentious issue in their relationship, which has contributed to the stress in Bob's life.

Bob's been seeing Dr. Martin every three to four months over the last two years, and the appointments typically last 15 minutes. He has good health insurance, so he can afford the doctor visits, lab tests and medications. Dr. Martin has started Bob on a variety of medicines, but his blood pressure and blood sugar are not controlled to the optimal levels, and he has not been able to lose weight despite her urging.

Bob likes Dr. Martin but is getting frustrated with his chronic health problems and hearing bad news at every check-up. He also hates taking the prescribed medications, following a special diet and checking his blood sugars. In truth, he often misses his medication, eats the wrong things, and occasionally skips checking his blood sugars. Bob is thinking, *It's hopeless. I'll never be any healthier than I am now. These medicines don't work and with my schedule there's just no way I can follow the diet or exercise plan that Dr. Martin wants me to. Doesn't she realize that it's impossible? No one could do it, especially me.*

As his physician, Dr. Martin cares for Bob and wants to help him, but she likewise feels frustrated. Every time she sees Bob, Dr. Martin feels she's failing him because she knows that his illnesses are not controlled to the standards that her professional association recommends. She would like to spend more time with Bob than a short 15 minutes but it "just isn't possible" in today's busy medical practice. Dr. Martin is also starting to believe that Bob is part of the problem. She thinks, *Why won't he simply follow the diet and exercise recommendations I've made over and over? I really can't do anything more to help Bob if he won't help himself.*

The following summer, while Dr. Martin is on vacation, Bob sees her partner, Dr. Stone, for a routine visit. Dr. Stone discovers that Bob is on some older medicines and hasn't had all of the recommended lab tests for his conditions. He makes a few changes for Bob and things get slightly better for a short while, but unfortunately they quickly revert to "normal." When Dr. Martin gets back, she's embarrassed about having overlooked the lab tests and not having considered a change to some of the newer medicines. She vows to try harder to keep up with the latest recommendations for the treatment of diabetes and high blood pressure.

This pattern goes on year after year without any meaningful improvement in Bob's health. In fact, the opposite occurs. Now age 55, Bob develops even more severe medical problems from his uncontrolled diabetes and high blood pressure. He is seeing Dr. Martin every other month, and has gained another 17 pounds. At 57 pounds overweight, he can't even walk a city block due to his obesity, advancing heart disease and numbness in his feet. He's on six medicines a day now, up from three when this story began, and all of his "numbers" are worse.

The next ten years are not good ones for Bob. His life begins to be dominated by his medical problems. He sees Dr. Martin monthly for routine visits and urgent problems that happen all too frequently. Bob develops severe heart disease in addition to chronic kidney failure, major nerve damage in his arms and legs, and, of course, even more poorly controlled diabetes and high blood pressure. He is now experiencing chest pain once or twice per week. At the age of 62, he requires two coronary angioplasties followed by open-heart surgery. These help for a while, but after just three more years, he dies suddenly at age 65 of a massive heart attack.

Wait a minute, what happened here?!

Everyone's intentions were good. Bob wanted to get better, and Dr. Martin wanted to help him. *Bob got a full dose of traditional healthcare; however he gradually got worse, felt terrible, and died too early!* Yes, it's true that the care he received slowed the progression of his illnesses compared with doing nothing, but it certainly can't be called a success.

Over the course of the story, both Bob and Dr. Martin felt frustrated but both believed there was nothing more they could do to change things for the better. Gradually they accepted the situation as the best that could be done and Bob progressed through a long slow decline to an early death.

Perhaps you think this story is a little unrealistic, perhaps exaggerated for effect. I assure you it isn't. It didn't take too many years in practice for me to see this story, or one pretty similar, repeated over and over again. There are millions of Bobs and thousands of Dr. Martins all across America living out this unfortunate story every day. You may be Bob. *Really!* This is the day-to-day reality of many, if not most, primary care practices. Take this book with you on your next visit to the doctor's office and get her opinion about whether this is the "norm." In my experience, this is reality.

Why Did Bob Die Early?

Who's to blame for Bob's long decline and premature death? Should Bob's wife, Susan, blame Dr. Martin, since it was her responsibility to control Bob's medical conditions better? Should Dr. Martin believe that it was all Bob's own fault because he didn't follow her instructions? Rather than assigning blame, let's look instead at some factors that we covered in the introduction which contributed to this tragedy.

Both Dr. Martin and Bob himself defined Bob as "the patient" to be "fixed" by the doctor. Bob took limited personal responsibility for trying to correct his medical problems, partly because it's a hard thing to do, but also because our entire culture tends to support us in not accepting responsibility for our self-imposed health situations and their consequences. Many people seem to believe that medical problems "just happen" to them, independent of their actions, like the weather: sunny or raining, the weather just happens by itself. Of course, some medical problems do come "out of the blue," but the majority of chronic health issues afflicting Americans today are, in large part, attributable to their own behavior. Also, our culture tends to glorify the practice of medicine, which fosters the belief among most people that understanding and managing our own health is beyond our grasp and that doctors have all the answers to every problem—usually in the form of pills.

Dr. Martin knew she needed to spend more time with Bob to better explain his issues and her recommendations, but she felt she just couldn't do it. If she had, she might have learned more about Bob's home life and the stress he was under in his marriage and at work. Bob didn't have many friends or hobbies, and unfortunately one of the ways Bob "managed" his stress was with "comfort foods." The more stressed he became, the more he ate. He attained short-term relief at the expense of his long-term health.

When Bob saw Dr. Stone one time, a few things were changed for the better. It didn't help much in the long run with his underlying illnesses but it was a higher level of care. What happened here? Well, treating chronic conditions such as diabetes is

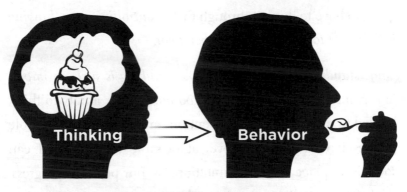

FIGURE 2.1   Thinking controls behavior.

them. But even these automatic behaviors started with thought and became automatic only through repetition.

A good example of an automatic behavior could be driving to your workplace every weekday. At first you had to learn the route, but after driving it many times, you don't really need to think about it at all. You just "drive to work." The proof that it's automatic comes on the occasional day that you're supposed to go somewhere else in the morning, but instead you drive to your workplace "without thinking."

This is important because *it is exactly some of those automatic behaviors that often result in negative health effects*. For example, eating food because it's in front of you instead of because you're hungry is a common ingrained and harmful behavior. Eating all that's served or "cleaning your plate" is another. You can probably think of many other examples.

The good news is that you can create new and beneficial automatic behaviors that you can use to your advantage, but you're going to have to think it through first. *Controlling your thinking is the secret to controlling your behavior.*

Understanding and controlling your thinking is such an important point that I cannot stress it too much! Our ability to think has led to wonderful ideas, inventions and almost unbelievable progress in healthcare. However, at the same time our minds can sometimes place artificial limitations on our personal progress. Without our realizing it, our thinking can trap us into views or mental models of reality that are false. As these thoughts or mental models become deeply ingrained, they begin to constitute our "worldview" which can be described as our personal mental perception of reality, or "how the world is." *Unfortunately, even widely accepted, culturally reinforced worldviews can be wrong.*

Thoughts Are Not Facts

Here are some examples. Up until the beginning of the 20th century, doctors *knew* that bleeding was a good treatment for many serious illnesses. Countless patients were harmed until doctors understood they were wrong. How many years did it take for most Americans to change their thinking about cigarette smoking, which at one time was portrayed as sophisticated and safe by docotors and athletes? Not until very recently have we learned that even being exposed to secondhand smoke can be quite harmful to our health.

Perhaps you *know* that it's *impossible* for you to lose weight. Unless you identify this as a *thought* and *not a fact*, you do not have an open mind and are not receptive to change. Your worldview of reality could be limiting you. I know that my own mental models have held me back over the years, which is why I'm so glad that I've learned to be wrong and to change. As Norman Vincent Peale put it, "Change your thoughts and you change your world."

Tame Your Ego

So, *in order to change your behavior, you must first change your thinking*. Sounds simple doesn't it? It *is* a simple idea, but doing it is often very hard. In order to change your thinking or point of view, you must first be willing to consider another point of view. How many arguments happen every day between people who cannot calmly and thoughtfully consider a different point of view? Democrats vs. Republicans, socialists vs. capitalists, creationists vs. evolutionists, vegetarians vs. meat eaters—the list is endless. You can see how these conflicts in thinking can lead to everything from a family argument at the dinner table to an armed conflict between nations.

Why do we find it so hard to change our thinking? In my view, it is *because we might have to admit we were wrong!* Oh no, not that again! *Yes, that!* Of course, we all must be wrong sometimes, but many of us would rather deny this and insist we're always right. That's why arguments seem more common than enlightening discussions among individuals with differing views. Very few people are really open-minded to such a degree that they will freely consider that they might be wrong on all kinds of issues. It's just too painful.

Often, people can't admit they're wrong unless there appears to be no other choice. Here's a personal example. At one time I had a fairly strong psychological need to be right. Consequently, I was somewhat arrogant, and could be argumentative and overly critical of others. This behavior alienated my boss and coworkers. Eventually things became so bad that my boss made it crystal clear to me that my behavior was a problem and it needed to change.

It wasn't a pleasant meeting. At first, I rejected this blunt feedback and looked for another explanation. The boss doesn't understand, I concluded. I even considered quitting because "they don't appreciate me here." But as I reviewed all the alternatives, thankfully, I decided to accept that my behavior *was* a problem, that I *was* wrong and that I needed to change. And I did change, becoming a more friendly, accepting and tolerant person.

How did I do it? *I learned it was okay not to be perfect.* Was it easy? No. Was it the right thing to do? Yes. I'm happy I was able to change my thinking and behavior rather than lose my position. This and other similarly jarring experiences in being wrong have taught me not to wait until there are no other options. *Instead, I try to actively look for areas where I might be in error and readily accept my mistakes in order to embrace new ideas.*

Just think about this for a while. It should be relatively easy for you to find an example from your own life experience. Perhaps you've had an argument with your spouse over who misplaced the car keys, the TV remote, or some other relatively insignificant item. Then you discovered that you were wrong and your spouse was right. How did it feel to know you were wrong? Not good, I imagine. Were you able to admit that to your spouse and even apologize? I hope you were, but many people are not.

Why does it feel so bad to be wrong? It hurts our self-images. We all have an "ego" which can be described as our sense of self, as distinct from others. Our egos seem to be constantly worried about what other people think of us, as if that were the sole determinant of our worth. We worry that if we're wrong we'll somehow be diminished or become less important in the eyes of others. While none of this is true, it sure feels that way at the time. But other people's opinions of you only have the importance that you give them in your own mind. *Free yourself from others' opinions of you.*

It is critical that you understand and appreciate this point, because *in order to get healthy, you're going to have to change your behavior. In order to change your behavior, you're going to have to change your thinking; and in order to change your thinking, you're going to have to get over your ego* (Figure 2.2).

Getting over your ego is not a one-shot deal; it's a process. The more you do it, the easier it gets. For now, just a little bit of dialing down your ego will go a long way (Figure 2.3). You don't have to be the most humble person on your block. You just have to be willing to be wrong and then to change your thinking accordingly.

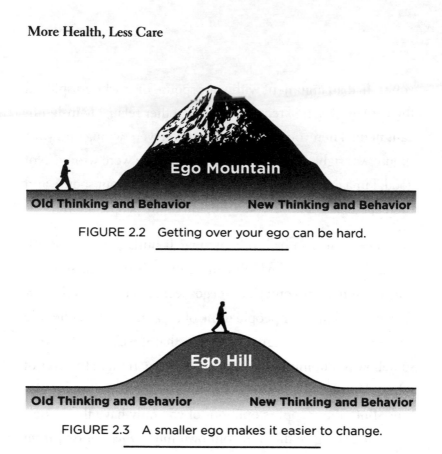

FIGURE 2.2   Getting over your ego can be hard.

FIGURE 2.3   A smaller ego makes it easier to change.

It might be comforting to realize that the ideas you're giving up probably weren't yours in the first place. You learned them from someone else at some point. For all you know, that "someone else" has since changed his mind about things too. Here's an example from my medical career.

In the first years of medical school I learned from my highly respected professors that intestinal ulcers are caused by "stress" and excess stomach acid. This was incorrect but they didn't know it at the time. By the time of my graduation, Australian physicians Dr. Robin Warren and Dr. Barry Marshall had identified that infection with the bacterium *H. pylori* is the true cause of ulcers. *Many of medicine's leading authorities immediately rejected this new (and true) idea.* Their minds were not open.

It took another ten years or so before Drs. Warren and Marshall were widely acknowledged to be correct in their findings. Later they were awarded the Nobel Prize in medicine for their discovery. I had to learn this new idea too, however my ego didn't have to be at stake if my professors had been wrong all along. Giving up the old idea was the right thing to do.

You can see that Bob and Dr. Martin never had any fresh ideas and so remained stuck in a pattern that really wasn't helping Bob. Dr. Martin continued to recommend diet and exercise plans that Bob couldn't or wouldn't adhere to, and Bob continued the same lifestyle that created his conditions in the first place. They needed to go find some new ideas and let go of old ones that weren't helping, but they couldn't do it.

The good news is that *you* can do it! Everything that I am telling you in this book I've had to learn for myself too. Hopefully I can make it a bit easier for you. Remember, I'm a doctor and big egos come with that professional territory! But also remember, I admit to being wrong a lot. (If you're in doubt, call my office and ask my staff about it.) Being wrong doesn't make me less of a person, and it won't hurt you either. Quite the opposite! It's an important and liberating step on your road to better health.

Now that you're ready for some new ideas, keep reading.

Personally I'm always ready to learn,
although I do not always like being taught.

SIR WINSTON CHURCHILL

CHAPTER THREE

Be Your Own Doctor: Preparing to Write Your Personal Prescription

As we learned from Bob's story, relying solely on traditional healthcare won't make you well. You have some specific health issues, and you want to be healthy. You must take charge of your own health and *be your own doctor*. (Maybe your mother always wanted you to be a doctor—now's your chance!)

I'm not suggesting that you opt out of traditional healthcare altogether. You still should have a personal physician and you may require other professional services too, but *you must be in charge*. Think of yourself as the lead doctor for your health and medical treatment team. In that spirit, here's what it takes to be a good doctor.

19

Be a Student of Health and Medicine

First, there's a lot of learning. College, medical school, and residency all require many years of study (13 years in my own case). Then you face continuing education, board certification, and researching difficult medical problems. Add it all up, and it represents a major commitment to lifelong learning. The best doctors are constantly learning new ideas and seeking out new information. You want to be the best doctor, since *you will also be the patient.*

Therefore, you need to be a lifelong student of health. The good news is that you aren't trying to be a brain surgeon at Harvard. You must only learn *just enough* to be a great doctor to yourself. How much do you know about your illnesses or your medications? Have you *seriously* studied health and wellness? Could your knowledge be too superficial? Are there new facts and ideas about health and wellness that could help you if you understood and applied them? Yes there are. My goal in this book is to get you started learning what *you* need to know. You *can* learn enough to help yourself, but you must make the commitment. What do you expect from your actual doctor? You wouldn't want to put your life in the hands of a physician who stopped learning ten years ago, would you?

Accept Responsibility and Make a Commitment

Second, a doctor *accepts responsibility* for the treatment of his patients. You'd be angry with a physician who agreed to treat

you today but changed his mind a few weeks fro...
the worst things a doctor can ever do is to aband...
who needs his help. In such a case, a doctor may be se...
ciplined by his state Board of Medicine, even to the poin...   ...os-
ing his license. If you abandon yourself, you won't lose a license,
but you will lose your chance to be healthy, and like Bob, you
could lose your life.

The doctor makes a commitment to treat the patient to the best
of his ability at all times and to help the patient find an answer.
A good doctor partners with his patient until a satisfactory solution is reached. He doesn't give up on the patient when things
aren't going well. Dr. Martin never actually gave up on Bob.
She just ran out of ideas, and wasn't willing to seek out new ones
that might have helped her patient. She accepted the *thought*
"nothing else can be done" as a *fact*.

Being your own doctor means that you will not give up on yourself and that you will accept personal responsibility for developing your own "prescription" for health and well-being. You
should never accept that "nothing else can be done" to improve
your well-being.

Be Honest and Courageous

Lastly, let's talk about honesty. A doctor needs to level with his
patients. This can be hard, as sometimes there are uncomfortable truths to be shared. It might be a confrontation about the
patient's behavior, such as excessive drinking. Or perhaps the

patient is dying and no one wants to talk about it. Unfortunately, some doctors will shy away from the hard truths. Here's an example.

Betty is dying of cancer, and more chemotherapy isn't going to help. She and her husband Keith prefer to ignore the obvious severe deterioration in her condition and always ask the caregivers to "do everything possible to fight the cancer." Her doctor feels uncomfortable trying to broach the issue with Betty or her husband that her death is imminent and that further chemotherapy will only be harmful. Consequently, he continues to order chemotherapy even though he thinks she can only live another month or two at best. Betty develops pneumonia and heart failure as a result of the treatment and spends the last three weeks of her life in the hospital unconscious and on a ventilator. Her grown children fly in to visit only after she has lapsed into a coma.

Here's how it could have gone:

Betty is dying of cancer, and more chemotherapy isn't going to help. Her doctor feels uncomfortable prescribing further chemotherapy knowing that it won't help and will likely harm Betty. He knows that she probably only has one to two months to live and is concerned that she not spend it severely ill. He schedules a quiet moment with Betty and Keith and is completely honest with them about the situation. It is difficult at first but through caring, honesty and persistence over several days he helps them see the harm in any further chemotherapy and the benefit of hospice care.

Betty decides to have hospice care at home and her children fly in from around the country to be with her. Over the next three weeks they talk, laugh and cry together as they reminisce about her life and say their goodbyes. Betty is awake and not in too much discomfort right up until the last day of her life. On that day she is asleep from the pain medicine and passes away peacefully surrounded by her family. Keith and the children are grateful for the final days they spent with Betty.

Which is the better outcome? Although Betty would never regain her best health, by facing reality with courage she and her doctor were able to create better health and well-being at the end of her life.

Perhaps you're thinking, "Why is he talking about that? Certainly as my own doctor, he's not expecting me to tell myself that I have incurable cancer!" That's true, but *being honest with yourself about your problems can be very difficult* — just as difficult, if not more so, than the hard conversations that come up in the practice of medicine. It's hard, but "Dr. You" is going to have to level with "Patient You" about your problems. We'll talk more about this later.

Okay, so far, so good. Hopefully, you're feeling like maybe you can be your own doctor, and you can be a good one. You can. But what kind of *patient* are you going to be? The doctor and the patient must work together for a good outcome. The commitment needs to go both ways. You *can* be a great doctor for yourself, but "Dr. You" is also looking for a great patient.

Honesty is the first chapter of the book of wisdom.

Thomas Jefferson

CHAPTER FOUR

Be a Great Patient:
Four Must-Have Attributes

Sometimes it can be pretty frustrating being a doctor. Think about how Dr. Martin felt all those years trying to help Bob improve his health. It was a losing battle. But, every once in a while, a doctor helps a great patient *really* get well and that makes up for a lot of frustration. Usually it's when the patient takes an active role in improving. The four "must have" attributes of a great patient are acceptance of responsibility, willingness to learn, honesty, and commitment to getting better.

Responsibility

Yes, the patient has responsibilities, too. Dr. Martin was responsible for trying to help Bob, and she did the best she thought

25

she could do, but Bob was the one with the illness. Bob was responsible whether he accepted it or not. The patient must accept responsibility and be the "owner" of the problem and its resolution. How can it be otherwise? You can change doctors three times, but the problem stays with *you*, the patient. Like Bob, you *have* the responsibility for your health, and the question is *do you accept it*? Accept *total responsibility* for your own health. The doctor is your partner in health, not the boss.

Please note that I am *not* saying that the patient is responsible for having an illness, problem or for the shape that she's in now. This is not about blaming the patient or anyone else for the situation. *"Blaming" is never helpful in problem solving.* You just need to take responsibility for improving yourself from today forward.

This idea of taking personal responsibility for individual health problems is a polarizing issue for our society. Similar to other social problems, such as poverty, we often see two opposing views in public discussions of the matter. One view suggests that people's problems are their own personal responsibility in the blaming sense of "it's their own fault." This implies that nothing can or should be done to help those with such problems, because "it's up to them to change." The other view suggests that cultural and environmental forces cause people to have problems and it is in no way their own responsibility. This implies that the individual need do nothing about his own problems because it's up to society to change and solve the problems for him.

There's an element of truth in both views. Cultural and environmental forces definitely help to create issues such as the epidemic of obesity as well as other social problems, but society cannot ultimately solve an individual's problem. An individual must take personal responsibility for solving his own problem, but he may need some help from others in actually doing so. As a society, without placing blame, we should invite individuals to take personal responsibility for addressing their health problems, while recognizing that the culture and environment may have played a large role in the development of the problems. Of course we should also provide the help and support they will require to improve.

Your particular problems may or may not be considered "your fault" by yourself or others. Perhaps you consciously chose to start smoking, and now you can't seem to quit. Or perhaps you really do have "bad genes" and your entire family has been seriously overweight for generations. Or perhaps your dysfunctional childhood played a role in your anxiety and depression now. Ultimately, it really doesn't matter! *What matters is accepting total responsibility for improving your health starting now.* Blaming yourself, the environment or anybody else for your health problems is a way to *avoid* responsibility. Blaming will keep you stuck where you are. Don't fall into that trap.

No one else will care about your health more than you. No one else will suffer the consequences of your health problems more than you. No one else will reap more benefit from your solutions than you. It *is* all about you. And you *are* ultimately in charge. The good news is that you don't have to go it alone. Later, we'll discuss how to get the help you'll need.

✔ REALITY CHECK

Please check one box.

❑　I accept personal responsibility for my health.

❑　I don't accept personal responsibility for my health.

I hope you checked the first box. If you checked the second, guess what? *You're Bob!* Please start over at Chapter One.

Willingness to Learn

Now that you're ready to assume total responsibility for your health, it's time to learn something about it. A great patient works with his doctor to help implement her recommendations. The patient needs to learn about his illness, his medicines, and how to change his lifestyle in order to be healthier.

How much learning do you need to do? You might already know a great deal about diet and exercise. Many people think they do simply from exposure to popular media. However, short media sound bites or news blurbs often oversimplify complex issues. More importantly, most people don't know enough about the deeper issues fundamental to lifestyle change, such as how to manage their own attitudes and emotions and how to effectively change habits.

Don't trust that you know enough. You don't. Be willing to learn more. You don't have to be a walking encyclopedia on health and diseases, but you must learn enough to help yourself and you *can* do that. An ill-informed patient has not truly accepted responsibility for his own health.

Honesty

Just as a good doctor needs to be honest with the patient, a great patient is honest with his doctor. Many times in my career, it's taken many visits for the truth to come out from patients about embarrassing or difficult subjects. Months or years may have gone by before a patient was honest with me about how much he drinks, about missing the medication, or about failure to follow through on an important part of treatment. Perhaps you too have not "fessed up" to something the first time the doctor has asked you about it. In any event, I am sure that you know from your own experience that it is often very hard to admit to an error or problem. Like we discussed, the ego doesn't like it. However, if you are going to be a great patient, *you are going to need to be honest with yourself.*

Oftentimes being honest with yourself isn't all that easy, as I mentioned after the story of Betty and her family in the last chapter. Unfortunately, denial can intervene. Denial is an ego defense mechanism in which the mind suppresses uncomfortable thoughts about difficult issues or facts. Because it's so common, we'll talk about how to avoid denial later. Honesty may not be easy but it is essential.

Commitment to Health

Lastly, let's talk about a commitment to getting better. Commitment is a strong word and a powerful motivator. Without it you're not going to be a great patient. A commitment is a binding obligation to a course of action. Some common examples of major life commitments are getting married, taking a mortgage to purchase a house, and enlisting in the military. Each of these commitments is made with a typical ceremony or protocol and a binding written document. Your commitment needs to be just as serious. Once you are committed to health and wellness there is no turning back.

Not everyone is willing to commit to getting well. Some patients actually seem to like their illnesses and welcome the special attention they get from being sick. Most people aren't like this. They want to get better. But when the going gets tough, they just can't seem to do what it takes to improve—like Bob who just couldn't manage to lose the excess weight that was the cause of his diabetes. Whether we admit it or not, we all have a lot of Bob in us.

If you want to be a great patient, you will need to make a lasting commitment to be healthy. As we discussed above, commitment doesn't mean just deciding to be healthy on a whim, or after a few minutes thought, or after two glasses of wine. Committing means deciding to be healthy after careful and prolonged reflection on the seriousness of the problem and then obligating yourself to follow through with action.

Too many people are casual in their decision to become healthier, giving no more time to this big decision than they do to selecting an outfit to wear in the morning. Casual or quick decisions like this are easily made and easily rescinded. A New Year's resolution is a good example of a *decision* to be healthy that usually isn't backed by a *commitment* to be healthy.

You must seriously decide to change and be *totally committed* to that decision including the actions and consequences that will follow from it. Think of deciding on your mate, or your choice of career or whether or not to have children. These are decisions with power and consequences. The decision to be healthy must be accompanied by a similar life-changing commitment. You must be ready to do *whatever it takes* to carry out your decision to be healthy. Commit to being healthy for life!

Probably you have been too casual about this in the past. Most people have had this experience. This time it needs to be different. I suggest that you meditate or pray about your decision. You might wish to seek help from supportive friends or relatives. Ask them to encourage you and be willing help you keep your commitment to yourself. Visualize your future lean and healthy body. Feel the energy of your good health to come. *Make the commitment.*

I'm about to ask you to formally make this commitment to yourself, but before I do, let's briefly discuss *setting goals.* Goals are important, but there are divergent views on exactly how best to choose a goal. Some experts emphasize a step process, suggesting that many sequential easily met "mini goals" are better than one big hard to reach goal. Others disagree. Almost everybody agrees that specific and measurable objectives with a due date are better than those that are "fuzzy" or ill-defined and open-ended.

Don't get stuck in that debate here. At this point, you may not be knowledgeable enough to create an appropriate well-defined goal. In my experience a *commitment* to an admittedly fuzzy goal such as "to be healthy" is head and shoulders above a *decision* without commitment to a specific target such as "to lose 10 pounds in 3 months." It's fine for your goal to be more general as long as you make the commitment.

Get ready. Now, make this commitment. Take it seriously with this small ceremony and written agreement. When you are ready, complete the following statement. Be as specific as you can right now. Be personal. Be real. Write it out and sign it to demonstrate your commitment to yourself. Speak the statement aloud, and perhaps share it with a close friend.

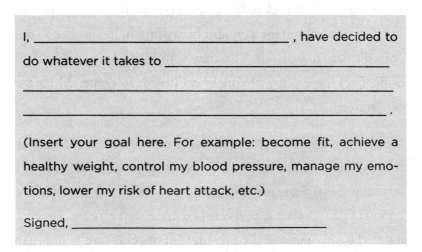

I, _____ , have decided to

do whatever it takes to _____

_____

_____ .

(Insert your goal here. For example: become fit, achieve a healthy weight, control my blood pressure, manage my emotions, lower my risk of heart attack, etc.)

Signed, _____

Congratulations on your success! How can I say that? Well, by committing to yourself to truly do whatever it takes to achieve your goal, you have guaranteed your eventual success. *Just keep at it.*

Summary

You probably have noticed that the responsibilities of the doctor and the patient are very similar:

Doctor	Patient
Accepts responsibility to help the patient.	Accepts responsibility for his own health.
Makes a commitment to help the patient to the best of his abilities.	Makes a commitment to do whatever it takes to be healthy.
Is honest with the patient.	Is honest with the doctor.
Is always learning the best medical practices.	Is always learning about his own health and illnesses.

With these mutual responsibilities in mind, let's go back to the story of Bob and think about it again. Bob thought of himself as a good patient. Dr. Martin thought of herself as a good doctor. Yet, together they participated in a decades-long relationship where Bob got slowly worse and died earlier than he should have.

Consider these questions:

- Did Bob accept responsibility for his own health?
- Was Bob ever honest with himself about his role in his own illness?
- Was Bob completely committed to getting well?
- Was Dr. Martin ever honest with herself that her efforts to help Bob weren't really working well enough?
- Could Dr. Martin have spent more than 15 minutes with Bob at his appointments?
- Was Dr. Martin completely committed to helping Bob get well?
- Did Bob or Dr. Martin learn all they could about other approaches, which might have helped?
- And most importantly, *How come nobody did anything differently?*

Bob and Dr. Martin learned to accept the situation the way it was, because to do otherwise *they would have to admit that they were wrong* (at least in part). It was just too painful to their egos for them to admit the truth. Bob could have admitted, "I haven't taken responsibility for my own health. I created my problems with my habits and I can solve them by changing my habits. If I can't do what Dr. Martin recommends, I've got to find something else that I can do. Other people have changed. I can too." Dr. Martin could have admitted, "What I'm doing to help Bob isn't working. There must be an answer, and we need to find it. I'm going to have to do something different." Instead they both participated in a relationship where it was understood that "this is the best we can do." It was easier on the egos involved.

Bob *was* ultimately responsible for his health. If Bob could have accepted responsibility, been *honest* with himself about his deadly lifestyle and followed the Personal Prescription for health, he would be alive, energetic and active today.

Commitment is what transforms a promise
into reality. It is the words that speak boldly
of your intentions. And the actions which speak
louder than the words. It is making the time
when there is none. Coming through time after
time after time, year after year after year.
Commitment is the stuff character is made of;
the power to change the face of things. It is the
daily triumph of integrity over skepticism.

ANONYMOUS

PAUSE FOR REVIEW

The concepts we've covered thus far are a critical foundation for what is to come. Let's pause here to review the building blocks that we've covered so far.

1. **Get ready**

   Relying on traditional healthcare is not enough.

   Change your thinking.

   Admit you may be wrong.

2. **Be your own doctor**

   Commit to learning about health for yourself.

   Take responsibility for writing your own prescription.

3. **Be a great patient**

   Accept total responsibility for your own health.

   Be honest with yourself about your health issues.

   Commit to do whatever it takes to improve your health.

Congratulations! By coming this far you are demonstrating the motivation and commitment to get healthy. Keep reading.

CHAPTER FIVE

Make a Diagnosis:
What's Wrong with Your Health?

Diagnosis: A Fancy Word for "Illness"

Now that you are committed to helping yourself, you need to better understand your medical issues and their underlying causes. Doctors call this a "diagnosis." (The term "diagnosis" is used to describe both the *process* of determining the cause/illness and the *actual* cause/illness itself) It's not too hard, but there are some finer points that we need to cover.

Start by assessing your symptoms (what you feel) and problems. These are the most apparent signs that something is wrong. However, symptoms and problems do not necessarily make a diagnosis, which is used to describe the underlying disease

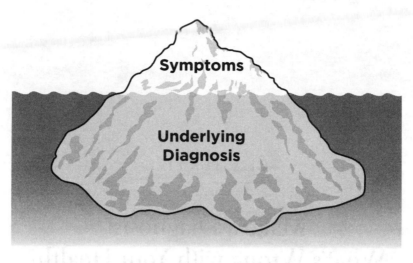

FIGURE 5.1   Symptoms can be just the tip of the iceberg.

process. (Figure 5.1.) For example, a patient might have knee pain and swelling (symptoms/problems) due to an underlying diagnosis of arthritis. However, the same or similar symptoms may arise from different underlying causes. In this example, the knee pain and swelling could also result from an infection or injury.

As other examples, fatigue (tiredness), weakness and being short of breath with exercise are common patient symptoms reported to doctors in any busy primary care practice. These problems could result from any of many different diagnoses including heart failure, emphysema, anemia, or just poor physical conditioning. Obviously, the treatment of poor physical conditioning is very different from the treatment of a serious heart or lung disease. I'm sure you get the point. The symptoms are a start, but the doctor must *dig deeper* to determine what's really going on.

Often patients have multiple problems and multiple diagnoses, which may interact with one another. Also, there may be an underlying diagnosis behind a particular illness or set of diagnoses. It's important to get to the deepest level of causality in order to prescribe the right cure. In Bob's case, he had at least three diagnoses: diabetes, high blood pressure, and obesity. These conditions frequently occur together as part of a larger diagnosis—metabolic syndrome—which is one of America's most significant public health issues. Perhaps Bob also suffered with an emotional disorder, such as depression. This could have contributed to overeating and under-exercising, which then led to weight gain and the resulting metabolic syndrome.

You can see that it is critical for the doctor not to stop too early in the diagnostic evaluation. If he stops before getting to the root of the patient's problem, he may prescribe the wrong treatment with potentially disastrous consequences.

Okay—now it's your turn again. Think about what symptoms and health problems you may have. Remember that "Dr. You" needs to be completely honest with "Patient You" about the issues. *Admit your problems to yourself.* Once again, it sounds simple, but it is not easy. Admitting that you have a problem can be very threatening to the ego, especially if your own behavior plays a role as it does in so many medical problems. In fact, many people get stuck in the quicksand of denial because it is just too painful for them to admit that they have problems. This is so important it is well worth spending some time on the subject.

Unmask Denial

"Denial" is a term used to explain circumstances where individuals do not accept reality as seen by others, and thus "deny" the objective facts. This is thought to occur unconsciously as a psychological defense mechanism because the situation is too emotionally painful to acknowledge. The teenager with anorexia nervosa dying of starvation, who believes herself to be too fat, and the alcoholic who denies any problem with drinking despite it being obvious to others, represent two relatively common examples of denial. If you have ever seen this in a friend or relative, you know how dramatic this type of denial can be.

Most of us adopt a subtler approach. More commonly, you might refuse to think about the issue, which has been termed "denial of impact." That is, you just don't want to think about your weight, your marital problems or the chest pain you have when exercising. In the "back of your mind," you know that you have a problem but you try to ignore the situation by refusing to allow "the front of your mind" to dwell on the matter. When it comes up to your consciousness, you forcibly suppress it.

In other cases, you might admit to having problems, but use minimization, rationalization or justification to explain why the issues exist and why nothing needs to be done to correct them. This has been termed "denial of responsibility." Perhaps you need to lose 20 pounds to help your diabetes, but your thoughts minimize the problem: "I'm not really overweight. Twenty pounds isn't a lot. Just look at me compared to Marcia or Joe.

They're really overweight." Or you rationalize the issue: "Yes, I am overweight, but I've been like this all my life, and my parents were too. It's in my genes. This is just the way I'm meant to be." Or you justify the situation: "I know I should lose 20 pounds, but it just isn't possible with my exercise limitations."

I've spent some time on this because, believe me, *denial is real* and it's a *real problem*. Denial can be completely unconscious and it will sabotage your efforts unless you constantly guard against it. *It is critically important for your health that you be completely honest with yourself.*

✔ REALITY CHECK

Please check one box.

- ☐ I am always honest and have never been in denial about my health issues.
- ☐ Denial about health issues has been and could continue to be a problem for me. I'll need to guard against it.

I hope you checked the second box, which I think applies to nearly all of us humans. *The single most important practice in avoiding denial is acknowledging that it can happen to you.* On a positive note, the fact that you're reading this book is a good sign that you know you have health problems and are looking for a solution. Don't let denial stop you short of the solution. You *can* do it!

Identify Your Problems

Now let's get specific about your health problems. I'll define a "problem" very broadly as anything that prevents you from being in the best possible physical or emotional health. As we've discussed problems can be diagnoses in themselves or symptoms of a separate underlying illness. Don't worry too much about that for now. Let's just identify your health problems. The list of statements below represents the majority of the lifestyle conditions addressed in this book.

✔ REALITY CHECK

Check the boxes of any that apply to you.

❑ I am seriously overweight.
❑ I have diabetes.
❑ My blood pressure is too high.
❑ I am depressed.
❑ I really need to begin exercising.
❑ I am an emotional wreck.
❑ My bad cholesterol is too high.
❑ I don't know anything about health.
❑ I'm on too many pain pills.
❑ My good cholesterol is too low.
❑ I smoke.
❑ I'm out of shape.
❑ I worry too much.
❑ My energy level is low.
❑ I just don't feel good.
❑ I've got to get off my sleeping pills.

> ✔ **REALITY CHECK**
>
> ❑   Tension and stress are killing me.
> ❑   I probably drink too much alcohol.
> ❑   If I don't change, I will die early.
> ❑   I really have a big problem with _____.
> ❑   I've been ignoring _____.

Okay, I know that checking a few of those boxes doesn't feel good, but it's the first step. If you weren't able to come up with any problems, you may be a perfectly healthy specimen of humanity, or more likely you may be in denial.

A good way to overcome denial and begin to identify your problems is to *ask for someone else's opinion, and accept their answers at face value*. What has your doctor told you? Is your spouse worried that you'll have a heart attack or stroke? Have your children nagged you to quit smoking or begin exercising? Really listen to those who care about you. Don't explain why they're wrong or excuse yourself from acting on the feedback that they give you. Just accept it, and then you can change. This technique of asking others is so powerful that I recommend it for everyone.

And what do you know deep down that is hard to admit? Remember, denial is an ego-defense mechanism, so *if it hurts your ego to think about it, you're probably on the right track*. Go ahead right now and take a few minutes or longer to identify your problem(s). You may wish to say them aloud or write them down before continuing. By ignoring your damaged ego, it will bother you less and less.

Peel the Onion to Find the Cause

Now that you've identified your problems and they are open to review, it's time to probe deeper to find the cause of the problem so you can do something about it. The "Five Why?" technique can be helpful to get to the root cause of a problem or issue. In this technique the goal is to keep asking "Why?" as each layer of the issue is revealed. Like an onion, there may be many layers before you reach the core. Consequently in this technique you ask "Why?" *at least five times*. Here is how it works.

Bob has diabetes and high blood pressure.

Why?—Because he has metabolic syndrome.

Why?—Because he is overweight.

Why?—Because he does not exercise and eats too much.

Why?—Because he is "stressed out" and mildly depressed, and his previous attempts to lose weight by "willpower" alone have failed. (And also, because his thinking has been shaped by a culture that fosters weight gain and inactivity.)

Why?—Because he has never learned how to manage his emotions.

Why?—Because he doesn't understand how to effectively change his habits.

We just investigated the underlying reasons for Bob's illnesses. You can see that after a while it gets pretty complicated, and there isn't always a simple and clear chain of causation. You have to do your own investigation, and it may require admitting to more issues. You may need to ask many more than five "whys." Don't worry if it's not all neat and clean, just keep at it. The more causes you identify, the more chance you have to make an improvement that will last. Getting to the root cause(s) provides you with the very best chance of solving the issue. I strongly suggest that you do this in writing and be as thorough as possible before reading further in this book.

Here are some "becauses" which you may find helpful.

✔ REALITY CHECK

Check any that apply to you:

- ❑ Because I am overweight.
- ❑ Because I am so stressed out.
- ❑ Because my job is so demanding.
- ❑ Because I feel guilty.
- ❑ Because I like it.
- ❑ Because my friends do it.
- ❑ Because it hurts when I exercise.
- ❑ Because I am not really committed to _____.
- ❑ Because I don't know how to _____.
- ❑ Because my whole family eats that way.
- ❑ Because I don't have any friends.
- ❑ Because the food served at work is bad for me.

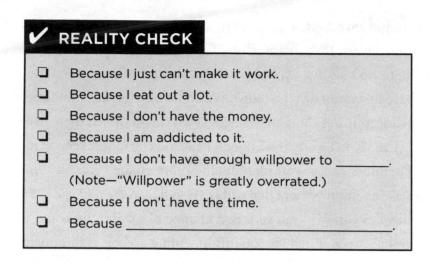

❑   Because I just can't make it work.
❑   Because I eat out a lot.
❑   Because I don't have the money.
❑   Because I am addicted to it.
❑   Because I don't have enough willpower to _____.
     (Note—"Willpower" is greatly overrated.)
❑   Because I don't have the time.
❑   Because _____.

Explanations Are Not Excuses

It's important to realize here that you are seeking to *explain* your issues, not *excuse* them. Explanations are concerned with the reasons why events happen, but excuses are used justify the appropriateness or necessity of events. Many of the statements above, and perhaps some of your own explanations, can be used as excuses if you're lacking commitment and seeking to let yourself off the hook for changing your behavior. Don't do that. Understanding how things got to be as they are, without accepting the explanation as an excuse, will help you design a health improvement program that will succeed where others have failed.

For example, when asked why he doesn't exercise, Roy replies with one of the statements above, "Because I don't have the money," meaning he feels that he can't afford to join a health club. Naturally, as Roy designs his program he should ask himself the following questions: "Do I really need to join a health club, or am I just using this as an excuse? What exercises could I do without joining a fitness center? Are there some deep discount gyms in town that I can afford? Could I save money somewhere else, perhaps cut back on dining out, to afford the health club that I think would be best for me?" And so on. You get the idea. Don't let an explanation become an excuse.

This exercise can be hard, not just because you may have to admit some uncomfortable truths about yourself, but also because it can sometimes be hard to break out of your own frame of thinking to see your particular situation from a different vantage point. It's easy to get stuck on an excuse. We've all done it.

If you seem to be struggling here, it may be helpful to have another person "interview" you on the issues. Let him or her ask the "whys" and record your answers, and perhaps ask some follow-up questions to clarify things and challenge you on any apparent excuses. Having to explain your answers to the "whys" as part of a conversation, and gaining the benefit of another's thoughts can allow you to see your issues from another perspective.

In fact, you may wish to use more than one person to refine your diagnoses and to get to the root causes before finalizing this list. Who are you going to use? We'll talk more about this in the next chapter.

One of the hardest things in this world is to admit
you are wrong. And nothing is more helpful in
resolving a situation than its frank admission.

BENJAMIN DISRAELI

CHAPTER SIX

Assemble Your Medical Team

Bob's Heart Surgery

Bob was about to have open-heart surgery. A nurse and an operating room technician had just helped him onto the operating table, where the anesthesiologist introduced himself. Over the next few minutes, the nurses and the anesthesiologist placed two intravenous lines and an arterial line into Bob's arms and hand. Simultaneously, he was "wired up" to the heart monitor and an oxygen sensor was placed on his finger. After a little I.V. sedative, Bob quickly fell asleep.

The anesthesiologist placed a breathing tube into Bob's throat and attached him to the respirator. Next, he placed a monitoring vascular line into the vein below the collarbone and threaded it through the right side of Bob's heart. Meanwhile the nurses had placed a catheter into Bob's bladder to remove urine and to monitor his core temperature throughout the surgery. Bob was then repositioned on the operating table, his skin was cleansed at the surgical sites, and sterile drapes were placed over the areas not involved. Bob was now ready for surgery.

With the operation about to begin, Bob was surrounded by the complete surgical team: the anesthesiologist at his head, the lead surgeon on his right, a nurse surgical assistant on his left, the scrub nurse at his right at thigh level and another surgeon across from her at Bob's left leg. In addition, the circulating nurse and other staff were in the room and ready.

Before beginning, every member of the team paused to verify that things were in order for this major procedure. The surgical plan was reviewed, sites were verified, and the various lines, devices and equipment were double checked until all members of the team agreed that nothing was amiss. Any member of the team could question anything that might be problematic, because all members of the team were responsible for making sure Bob's surgery went well.

No issues were identified and the operation commenced. Within minutes the surgical team was staring at Bob's beating heart. Working with the perfusionist who runs the heart/lung bypass machine, the primary surgeon carefully diverted the blood around Bob's hearth and through the machine. Although Bob's heart was beating, there was no blood flowing through it. The bypass machine had taken over.

Moving quickly, the surgeon paralyzed and cooled Bob's heart placing an iced saltwater solution into the sac surrounding it, and identified sites to place the vein grafts from the aorta to the coronary arteries. The second surgeon had the leg veins out and ready, and the three bypass grafts were placed without difficulty. An additional assistant had scrubbed in to hold the heart steady during this delicate procedure.

During this entire time, a constant stream of conversation was underway about the conduct of the operation—the two surgeons asking for instruments and assistance, the scrub nurse verifying their requests, various other staff reporting on their areas. And of course there had been constant physical cooperation among the team—the surgeons actually operating, the O.R. staff holding the heart, and the nurses handing instruments on and off and moving about the room as needed. Bob was at the center of a well-orchestrated performance by a talented cast.

Shortly after the bypass grafts were placed, the initial stages of the operation were carried out in reverse. Bob came off the bypass pump as his heart warmed and began contracting again. The sides of the chest were allowed to come together and the breastbone was wired closed. The skin was sutured, the drapes removed and Bob was moved to the recovery area to wake up from anesthesia. The operation was a success.

"Successful" Surgery = Failure of Personal Health

Yuck! Why are we reviewing Bob's bypass surgery? Two reasons: Number one is to give you the idea that you don't want to have this kind of operation. You can see the serious and risky nature of a procedure where doctors split open your chest, paralyze your heart and a machine pumps your blood. Things don't always go well in such operations. Some patients have complications. Some die.

Although it's true that the operation was a "success," the very need for the operation represents a failure. Bob could have avoided this major surgery and most of his other medical care. *A great deal of what we think of as "successful" medical care in America would be unnecessary if we would only live differently.* It's very ironic when you think about it. Our unhealthy American lifestyle has helped to create much of the need for high-tech medical care, which is in turn glorified in our popular culture.

The other reason for reviewing Bob's operation is that it provides a great example of medical teamwork for us to examine.

Teamwork: Essential for Success

The point here is that *doctors don't work alone.* I suppose that a doctor with a large ego could take sole credit for curing illnesses, but for any kind of serious medical care *it takes a team.* Bob's surgeons took special care in assembling their cardiac surgery team in order to get the best result. In fact most medical care similarly requires a team.

I am sure that you know this from your own experience with healthcare. Nurses, medical assistants, receptionists, laboratory technicians, X-ray technicians, physician assistants, nurse practitioners, pharmacists and other physician specialists may all be part of your medical team, even for a relatively minor illness. Without the team, the solo doctor can't do much.

You shouldn't work alone either. Few great accomplishments are the work of an individual by himself. Changing your habits and your health will be a great accomplishment. To ensure your success, you want and need a personal health team to help you get there (Figure 6.1).

Do you really *require* a team? *Yes, absolutely!* Remember, if change were easy you would have already done it on your own.

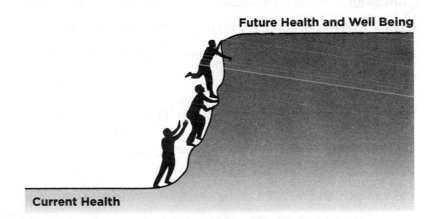

FIGURE 6.1   A team can succeed where one would fail.

A carefully selected health team will help encourage and support you as you navigate your journey to better health. Your health team can also help you with advice when you need it. *You can always benefit from listening to thoughts and opinions from someone who cares about you.*

What makes a team work well together? Think about the team for Bob's bypass surgery. The team members had individual areas of expertise, trusted each other, communicated well during the operation, and were all committed to a common goal: getting Bob through the operation successfully. During the operation no one was afraid to speak up or challenge another's thinking when there was a concern for Bob.

You need a team like this. In your case, the team won't always be working together at the same time and in the same place. In fact, one person on the team doesn't even need to know who else is on the team, as long as they are all helping you toward your goals. Your team members will help you evaluate information, test ideas, develop your plan and support you in its implementation. You are, like Bob's surgeon, the team leader.

Build a Winning Team

So, who should be on your health team? People you can trust, people who care about you and will help you succeed, and people with whom you can talk freely about personal issues. Your spouse or other family members may be a good place to start, but all families aren't loving, understanding and encouraging.

It's sad, but sometimes family members may even wish to see you fail because they are threatened by your desire to change. If your relatives are not supportive, then don't be afraid to forgo using family members. Only trusted family, friends and professionals *who encourage you* should be on your team.

How about friends from school, church or work? Most people have made at least one or two friends with whom they feel comfortable talking about personal issues. These are the friends you need. Remember the requirement for good communication; if you can't open up and share your struggles with your teammates, they can't help you.

Find Health Professionals That Fit

What about your doctor? Your doctor should be committed to helping you improve your health, but not every doctor is perfect. Be honest with your doctor about what you're trying to accomplish and ask for her help. Consider lending her this book and discussing the concepts as applied to your situation. A committed doctor should be a good source of health information and can help you sort out which ideas might be useful to you. Because she knows you and your health issues well, she should be able to help customize recommendations for your particular circumstances. For sure, she needs to be on your team.

However, not every doctor may be willing to work with you in the way that's best for you. Perhaps the doctor doesn't have enough time, doesn't communicate well, or dismisses your interest in alternative therapies and ideas. Physicians today are trained to focus much more on the treatment of disease than on how to help patients change. If things aren't going well with your doctor and you can't work it out to your satisfaction, it's okay to find someone new. This could be one of the most important decisions you will make, and you need the best help you can get on your team.

Also, seriously consider including a mental health professional, such as a psychologist or counselor, on your team. Psychologists have dedicated their careers to helping people change. They are professionals who are responsible for serving the best interests of their clients. Are you reluctant to see a mental health professional, even though deep down you think you might need one? Why is that? Perhaps it challenges your ego and you are worried about what others might think about you. Would you accept that in your doctor? What would you think of a doctor that wouldn't call a cardiologist in to help treat you during a heart attack because he was worried about his ego? *Don't be that kind of doctor.*

Remember how we began: thinking controls behavior. The ability to alter your thinking is the foundation for success in your Personal Prescription to health. This is what psychologists do: help people to change their thinking. Some people have such very ingrained thought patterns or worldviews that they are unable to break out of them on their own. Therapy or counseling simply helps them see new ideas and new ways of thinking, allowing them to grow and make positive changes in their lives.

You will be in good company if you decide to add a mental health professional to your health team. Tens of millions of Americans have sought help from a counselor, psychologist or psychiatrist. These are individuals with the courage to confront their problems and get better. It's just that few of them tell stories about their mental health therapy during the lunch break at work. Consequently, everyone thinks that "no one I know" goes for this kind of help. The truth is that lots of people do. I imagine that most were once reluctant to go, but now are glad they did. Also remember that *you have already decided to do whatever it takes* to be healthy. So if it takes seeing a mental health professional, *go for it*, and be proud of yourself! I will be proud of you.

If you're taking medicines, or considering taking them, a pharmacist could be helpful. A good pharmacist is able to help you understand the proper use of a medication including its potential side effects, interactions with food or other agents, and alternatives. A pharmacist can also be helpful in understanding natural or over-the-counter remedies, and may have more time available for you than most physicians.

Of course I've just named a few of the many types of healthcare professionals available to you. Depending on your individual needs, you may benefit from others on your team, for example, a podiatrist if you suffer from problems with your feet.

Consider a Coach

One specialist you should seriously consider using is a health and wellness coach. Personal coaching, an emerging field dealing with behavior change, can make a huge difference in your results. Health coaches are not trainers administering workouts or directing behavior. Think of them more as special advisors trained in helping you develop and achieve your own health and wellness goals. Typically coaches work through questioning, discussion and exploration, which help you to achieve greater focus and identify successful methods to change. Beyond conversation, the coach may suggest the client perform independent research or try new behaviors. The role of the coach is to help the client see new possibilities and successfully adopt new behaviors.

Having had a personal executive coach at work for several years, I've experienced the power of coaching. It really works! A good health coach could be the most powerful member of your team. I believe in the power of coaching so much that I have taken formal training in this area myself.

Because coaching is a relatively young field, it may be difficult to identify an appropriate individual in your area. Although many people may not be familiar with health coaching, I would still suggest you begin by asking around. Check with local health, wellness and fitness professionals for a recommendation. Also, the International Coaching Federation's (ICF) web site (www.coachfederation.org) has a helpful coach locator function.

Standards are evolving in this discipline and it is prudent to ask a prospective coach for references from prior clients. Look for training from an ICF accredited program. Certification from the ICF is a meaningful credential in the coaching field but still relatively uncommon. Interview several coaches before settling on the one for you. Importantly, coaching is not the practice of medicine or psychology. Your health coach should not attempt to diagnose or treat mental or physical illness.

Seek a Support Group

If you identified some form of addictive behavior as part of your diagnosis, you may wish to consider a 12-step program. I know I might be making some of you uncomfortable here, but keep an open mind. Others may be asking, "What's a 12-step program?" These are programs for people who share a common addictive illness and work together to help each other find ways to recover. Alcoholics Anonymous is the original 12-step group. Its success has led to the formation of other groups using similar methods, such as Overeaters Anonymous. Members commit to be on each other's teams and to helping each other get better.

In fact, at an Alcoholics Anonymous meeting it's exceedingly common for members to attribute their successful recovery to assistance from the other members of the group, *and they really mean it*. The value your team adds can be the difference between success and failure.

Other illness-specific support groups may be of value to you. For example, an arthritis support group or a group of cancer survivors. Support groups can be a great place to find team members who are familiar with your particular illness, problem or condition, and part of the whole reason to have a team is for support. Having some friends who have previously been through what you are currently experiencing can be very helpful, *as long as they are focused on helping you get better.*

A word of caution about support groups: not all groups are the same. Be careful not to join a support group where the members seem to derive their whole identity from having the illness or condition. There are some individuals who seem not to want to get better, but rather to enjoy being a member of the "sick club." You can identify them by their blaming and "victim mentality." Steer clear of people and groups like this. *Remember, your goal is better health, not validation for being ill.* Anybody that is going to be part of your team needs to be focused on your goal too, *getting better* no matter what illness or condition you have.

God As a Team Member

How about God? Should God be on your team? Perhaps you're thinking—"Wait a minute; I didn't think that this was a religious book. I just want to get healthy." Relax, this isn't a religious book. But you might want to think about these questions. Remember how we started: the first steps are to question your own knowledge and to change your thinking.

First let me acknowledge that "God" is a loaded term. It means many different things to different people. For our purpose here, when I use "God" I mean a loving and caring intelligence that is ultimately responsible for the seen and unseen world in which we live.

I obviously don't know what you believe about God, because we haven't met. You may be a Christian, a Jew, a Muslim, or a follower of another religion. Or perhaps you're agnostic or an atheist. We have to work out our own spirituality for ourselves, and I don't wish to advocate for any particular religious tradition here. But I *believe* that God loves all of us and wants to help us with our lives. If that is true, God qualifies to be on your team.

I also believe that you can communicate with God by praying. During your upcoming journey to good health I would recommend that you pray for guidance, insight, wisdom, strength, patience, determination and success in your quest. If you are not sure if God is real or is interested in you, I recommend praying for answers to those questions as well, and I also suggest that you discuss it with the people on your team. Belief in God isn't necessary for self-improvement, but it sure can help.

Take a minute now to identify potential team members.

My Potential Team Members

Friends

_____

_____

_____

Family

_____

_____

_____

Professionals

_____

_____

_____

Others

_____

_____

_____

Accept All the Help You Can Get

How big should the team be? Well, it's hard to answer that, but there is no shame in accepting help. In general I believe that bigger is better as long as the members meet your criteria. Think back to our cardiac surgery example. The cardiac surgery team had so many members because each provided a unique specialty or service that was needed in support of the overall goal of getting Bob off the table alive after a successful operation. You may need some additional specialists too—perhaps a personal trainer, chiropractor, dietician or nutritionist, clergyman, or dentist. The more team members, the more resources you have available to help you achieve health and well-being.

That said, don't be afraid to start small. Enlisting even one really close friend can make an enormous difference. If creating a large team sounds too scary or just doesn't resonate with you, I would suggest that you start with just two or three people on your team besides yourself. (And don't forget about considering a counselor and God.) You can approach these individuals, explain what you are trying to accomplish and ask them to encourage and support you along the way. It may help to give them a copy of this book so they understand what you're looking for. Adding people to your team slowly over weeks, months and years is a strategy many people use, and you may find it easy to expand your team once you've got the first one or two people on board.

People who work together will win, whether
it be against complex football defenses,
or the problems of modern society.

Vince Lombardi

PAUSE FOR REVIEW

Once again, let's pause to review and reinforce what we've covered so far. Take some time to reflect on these points.

1. **Get ready**

   Relying on traditional healthcare is not enough.

   Change your thinking.

   Admit you may be wrong.

2. **Be your own doctor**

   Commit to learning about health for yourself.

   Take responsibility for writing your own prescription.

3. **Be a great patient**

   Accept total responsibility for your own health.

   Be honest with yourself about your health issues.

   Commit to do whatever it takes to improve your health.

4. **Make a diagnosis**

   Identify your problems and their causes.

   Avoid denial.

5. **Assemble your team**

   Pick people who can really help.

   Build a strong team. Now!

   Include professionals and consider God.

So far, so good. There's just a little more to it.

CHAPTER SEVEN

More On Thinking:
Our Deadly Culture

You're almost ready to write your own prescription for good health, but before you do let's revisit your thinking and your ability to accept new ideas. Remember your mind is all-important for behavior change. If the mind is right the body will follow. Unfortunately, this is not as simple as you might think.

You may believe that thinking is pretty straightforward—after all, you've been thinking all of your life. You have a good brain and you know how to use it. Of course you do, but the point is that there are many important influences on your thinking and decision-making that are not so obvious (Figure 6.1). Do a little research of your own on the topic of denial that we covered earlier. Also, what influence does our culture have on your

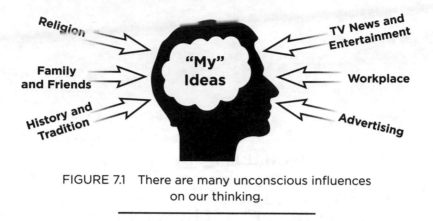

FIGURE 7.1   There are many unconscious influences
on our thinking.

thinking? What ideas do you believe just because you live in America in the 21st century? Are they all correct? Are they good for you?

This is critically important. Remember, you are going to become healthy by changing your behavior. And your behavior comes from your thinking, which in turn is very definitely influenced by our culture and environment. Typically, cultural influences are not overt "thought control," but instead imperceptibly shape our mental models of reality or worldviews. You need to explore these unconscious influences upon your thinking in order to prevent old ideas from holding you back. Here are some examples of what I mean about the effects of our culture and environment on our thinking.

Don't Be Brainwashed

Contemporary America is built on a foundation of consumerism, which is the idea that progressively more consumption of goods is good for society. Most advertising is designed to get us to consume more by making us think that buying more things is the way to personal fulfillment. It's not unusual to see ads that suggest that it is "good for the soul" to buy this brand of luxury car, or that "you have arrived" if you purchase that expensive wristwatch. With time, these ideas settle into your unconscious mind, becoming part of your worldview and often lead you to the "rat race," working harder and harder in order to buy more and more things, thinking that they will fulfill you.

The person caught up in a consumption-driven lifestyle may experience a great deal of stress. He would like to work less and live a more balanced lifestyle, but he won't be able to do it unless he gives up the unconscious consumerist views that he has adopted. Until then, he will feel that he doesn't have time for a more balanced lifestyle—working out, getting a full night's sleep, meditating, spending more time with family and friends. Or he might feel that money is too short to be spent on a fitness center membership, a vacation, or healthier food choices.

What do we consider beautiful or normal in a person's body? The American media has fostered the development of an ideal body image that often revolves around being unnaturally thin. Our culture also tends to glorify beauty and create idols of beautiful and quite slim individuals. This leads some normal healthy individuals, mostly young women, to strive to be unnaturally thin in the name of being beautiful. Simultaneously, in our everyday life we are surrounded by so many overweight individuals that being overweight is becoming the new "normal." The person who holds the view that being moderately overweight is "normal" is not motivated to lose weight.

Americans also cherish a cultural norm of rugged individualism. Think of "the Marlboro Man" or Rambo or many of Clint Eastwood's movie characters. These cultural icons suggest that we can be strong, independent and successful, no matter what the odds, and that being dependent on others is a sign of weakness. In reality, as we've already discussed in Chapter 6, everyone needs help. *You will have a much easier time in life if you can learn to ask for and accept help from others.*

In many respects, American culture worships high-tech medicine. Medical shows make for great nighttime dramatic TV entertainment. Glowing reports of the latest medical advances sell newspapers. Heart surgeons are always popular cocktail party guests. Doctors, patients and hospitals often seem fixated on the most modern, most expensive, and the most high-tech treatments and diagnostic tests, while ignoring what people need most, which is help getting healthy. Diabetes, for example, is defined as a "medical problem" and not as a "behavior problem" or "lifestyle problem," even though for the majority of diabetics a change in lifestyle could eliminate the diabetes.*

In addition, our culture suggests that fixing such medical problems is the doctor's job. The person who thinks that all of his problems are "medical problems" to be solved by doctors or medicines isn't likely to initiate the fundamental changes in per-

---

* Type II diabetes. See footnote on page xvii for more explanation.

sonal behavior necessary for good health. *It was this kind of thinking that killed Bob.*

Don't get me wrong. I love America and am grateful to live here. All cultures everywhere influence the thinking of the local people, and there is certainly a lot to like about our American culture. Freedom, respect, tolerance, and opportunity are hallmarks of America and make this a great nation. However, regarding health effects, our culture is not helping most of us.

These ideas can be hard to grasp. It may be difficult to accept that many of your beliefs arise from your environment, but I think you can see the truth of it through these few examples. The essential point is not to renounce your entire worldview immediately. It's enough to hold your beliefs lightly; be a little bit suspicious of your views about how things are. Trust the common knowledge less and give more effort to reasoning through issues for yourself. Be willing to think differently.

Okay, you're ready to examine your own thinking. Let go of any preconceived ideas and make a change for the better. Now you're ready to write your own prescription for health and well-being.

He who joyfully marches in rank and file
has already earned my contempt. He has been
given a large brain by mistake, since for him
the spinal cord would suffice.

ALBERT EINSTEIN

CHAPTER EIGHT

Write Your Personal Prescription

I hold a vivid memory of the time I wrote my first prescription as a newly graduated doctor. It was a very exciting and very scary experience all at the same time! As a brand new graduate, I didn't have a lot of experience and I was worried about getting something wrong and causing harm to the patient. I double and triple-checked to make sure I prescribed the right medicine at the right dosage. Fortunately, I did get it right and the patient did well. There's a lot that goes into selecting the proper prescription, but don't worry—you *can* write a prescription for good health that is just right for you.

You're Unique: Personalize Your Prescription

Every patient is unique, and every prescription must be tailored to the special needs of that individual. Some things a doctor considers before deciding on a particular prescription for a patient include:

- **Efficacy.** Is this a powerful medicine or a weak one? How likely is it that this medicine will actually work for this patient?
- **Side effects.** What, if any, side effects are possible with this medicine? Which are likely to occur in this patient? How bad would it be for this patient if those side effects actually developed?
- **Compliance.** How often does this medicine need to be taken? How big are the pills? Will the patient actually be able to take this medicine as directed?
- **Cost.** Can the patient afford this medicine? Are less expensive alternatives available?

After making a diagnosis and researching treatments, a good doctor attempts to select an affordable prescription medicine that is likely to work with no or minimal side effects on a reasonable dosing schedule. Usually there are lots of alternative choices and no one "perfect" treatment. All of the factors must be balanced against one another in making a choice that is good for the patient. Even a very powerful drug won't help if the patient can't afford it, or if it must be taken twelve times a day. In that case, a combination of two less powerful, but inexpensive, once-a-day pills might be preferred.

Now it's time to write your own prescription for better health and well-being. No one can tell you exactly what the right action plan to achieve better health is for you. You must figure it out yourself with the help of your team. Oh sure, people will tell you that you have to exercise more. But how often? Which exercises? Aerobics or weight lifting, or both? How long should your workouts be? These decisions are yours to make and you can do it. The first step is learning. And remember, you are committed to learning and welcome new ideas.

Take an Organized Approach to Learning

Take an organized approach to learning. Get a binder with dividers or several colored folders, one for each major topic of study. Initially your topics should include any health issues that you have identified, for example, diabetes and high blood pressure, as well as "health and wellness" in general. As you begin to acquire general knowledge, you will find yourself wanting to dig deeper into more specific health issues. For instance, a new topic of interest might be "aerobics" or even a particular aerobic exercise such as power walking. Start a new folder or binder section for each topic and *stay organized*.

Begin learning by logging on the internet and visiting local or online bookstores. I recommend using books as a source for general or comprehensive health and wellness information and relying on the internet for more specialized disease-related information.

Valuable general and disease-specific information is available from the United States Department of Health and Human Services, the Centers for Disease Control and Prevention, the National Institutes of Health, the National Institute of Mental Health, the National Library of Medicine and the National Center for Complementary and Alternative Medicine.

Additionally, major medical centers and universities typically have useful web sites covering all major health topics. The Mayo Clinic and Harvard University's medical school are good examples. Specialty associations, such as the American Cancer Society or American Diabetes Association are good sources for learning in their respective areas of concern.

Of course, not all internet sites are reliable. Which ones are you going to trust? The web address suffix can be helpful to you here. The most common suffixes are ".gov" for government sites, ".edu" for university sites, ".org" for nonprofit sites and ".com" for commercial sites. As you might suspect, the commercial sites are built for commerce. They're trying to sell you something. Give the government, university and major nonprofit sites more of your time at first. As your knowledge builds, you will be better able to judge the reliability of information from less authoritative web sites. To get you started, I've included a list of websites that I consider authoritative in the Resources section at the end of the book.

Books and the internet are certainly not the only sources of good health ideas. Many health-related magazines are available. General health periodicals are often designed exclusively for a male or a female audience, while others specialize in specific subjects of interest to both genders such as running or cycling. Visit your local library and review what's available. Subscribe to one or two magazines that look helpful. It's great to have new ideas arriving in your mail every month.

And don't forget people as a source of helpful information and inspiration. Talk to your friends and acquaintances about what works for them. Reach out to others. Approach someone you believe to be healthy and ask them about it:

> "Tim, you seem to be in great shape. How do you do it?"

> "Jane, I remember you lost a lot of weight a few years ago and you've kept it off. How did you manage it?"

> "Betty, you always seem so calm and cheerful even when everything is going wrong. How do you stay so happy?"

You can learn a lot this way. Most people are happy to tell you about themselves, and you may find a team member or two in the process.

So, jump into it. Become a student of physical, emotional and spiritual health. If you really don't know where to start, take a look at any of these topics that seem interesting:

- Accepting new ideas
- Alternative medicine
- Aerobic exercise
- Alcohol, health effects

- Anger, health effects
- Anxiety, health effects
- Automatic behavior
- Caloric density
- Calisthenics
- Carbohydrates, proteins and fats
- Changing behavior
- Changing your mind
- Cognitive behavior therapy
- Commitment
- Creating new habits
- Cultural influences
- Denial
- Dietary fiber
- Ego
- Emotional effect of food
- Emotional health
- Environmental influences
- Five why? technique
- Food diary
- Friends/friendship, health effects of
- God
- Glycemic index
- Justification
- Learning new things
- Low carbohydrate diets
- Meditation
- Mental focus

- Mental models or mental paradigms
- Minimization
- Optimism
- Normal body weight
- Peer pressure
- Persistence
- Personal trainers
- Pessimism
- Pilates
- Preventive medicine
- Probiotics
- Portion sizes
- Positive psychology
- Positive thinking
- Prayer
- Rationalization
- Resistance exercise
- Root cause analysis
- Self esteem
- Structuring your life
- Sleep
- Spiritual health
- Stopping bad habits
- Television, health effects
- Variation in healthcare
- Veganism
- Vegetarianism
- Visualization

- Vitamin supplementation
- Walking
- Willpower
- Worldviews
- Worry, health effects
- Yoga

These are just some topics that you may wish to research as you prepare to write your own prescription. It's not meant to be an exhaustive list. My purpose is to stimulate your thinking and curiosity. Learn, and apply your knowledge. Start here if you want. *Start now.*

Making Sense of the Information

If you are the least bit serious about studying health issues, you will likely be overwhelmed with information. The same thing happens to doctors all the time. Don't worry. You don't have to know everything, just *enough*. Think about how many books about diet and exercise you've seen or heard of in the last few years—the Atkins Diet, the South Beach Diet, the Mediterranean Diet. And there are ten times more that you've never heard of. The really bad news is that they may all be recommending different diets or different workouts. Why is there such a diversity of approaches? Do any of them work?

It's hard to say. I believe that for the most part, yes, they all "work" for some people some of the time, but not for everyone—just like the medicines that we talked about above. Everyone is unique. The combination of factors that affect your health is unique to you. These include your physical factors, emotional factors, spiritual factors, social factors, and environmental factors. Let's think about how these factors might combine in a whole person, and how health prescriptions might need to be different for different individuals. For example:

> Joan is a 66 year-old widow who lives with her sister in Ft. Lauderdale. She has weakness of the legs from polio as a child and has a hard time walking. She loves to swim, but hasn't done it much since her husband died a year ago. He used to drive Joan to the community pool. She is sad most of the time and eats more than she should. She is now 20 pounds overweight and has "pre-diabetes." Money is a little tight.

> Brad is 33, single and works in a high stress job on Wall Street. He gets to work at 7:00 A.M. and usually stays until 7:00 P.M. five days a week. He frequently works half days on weekends as well. He is happy in general and loves his job despite the long hours. He is thin, but he eats a lot of "junk food" and smokes a pack of cigarettes per day. He says that he has "plenty of money," but "no time" to get healthy.

> Beth is 26, married and a mother of two young children. Her husband, who is in software sales, travels frequently, and she works full time as a receptionist at a law office in order to help ends meet. She reports feeling exhausted all the time, but particularly dur-

ing the long winters in Maine. She is overweight, and hasn't had any regular exercise since high school when she was on the cross-country team.

Can you see how their different life circumstances require different prescriptions for health and well-being for Joan, Brad and Beth? Here are the solutions they worked out.

Joan has a caring doctor who identified her sadness as early depression and recommended therapy. Although initially reluctant and wary of the expense, Joan decided to see a counselor and work through her grief. As her mood improved, she and her sister decided to seek out new friendships among women from their church and the condominium in which they live. They now have a group of "Seven Sisters" who enjoy getting together socially and helping each other. Two enjoy water aerobics and Joan is now back at the pool with them three times a week. Her overeating seemed to "take care of itself" as her mood improved and she became more active, and she's lost 15 of the 20 pounds gained in the year after her husband's passing.

Brad worked with a health coach to develop his plan of action. He decided not to give up his busy lifestyle, but to use some of his money to compensate for his lack of time. In order to give up the junk food, he hired a personal chef to prepare meals for home and work. Every Sunday, his chef prepares six days' worth of delicious and healthy meals and stocks Brad's refrigerators for the coming week. (Brad purchased a small refrigerator for use at work.) He funds a supply of fresh fruit for his office, and his assistant keeps the bowl full of apples, bananas and other seasonal fruit. Brad found a fitness center two blocks from his office and works out for 45 minutes with a personal trainer at noon Monday, Wednesday and Friday. He's found that the personal trainer keeps his workouts very focused and intense, helping him to save time. Unfortunately Brad still smokes. He says that he "can quit cold turkey when I want to," but he hasn't decided to quit yet.

Beth spoke with her doctor, who found she had a mild iron deficiency and a mild case of seasonal affective disorder (SAD). He recommended an iron supplement and the use of a light therapy box, but he mentioned that light therapy was not actually approved by the Food and Drug Administration (FDA) for treatment of SAD. Beth started the iron supplement immediately and commenced light therapy a few weeks later after researching it for herself. Beth is now exercising on a treadmill and a stationary ski machine that she and her husband agree were excellent investments in her health. She feels great and is looking forward to getting back outside for running and skiing when the kids are a little older.

Joan, Brad and Beth each required a *personal* prescription. So too will your prescription need to be uniquely tailored just for you. Relax. You *can* do this.

Don't be afraid of the sheer volume of information out there. Keep learning. Take your time and think it through. Discuss new ideas and unfamiliar concepts with your team. As your knowledge expands, you will find it easier and easier to make sense of it all. *Keep at it.*

As you research ideas, *feel free to mix and match ideas from different sources*. You might like some of the ideas based on one approach and some from another. It's okay if you get only a single good idea from an entire book. That's one more idea to incorporate into *your* plan. You are *creating* something that will work for you, not *discovering* the exact solution.

Complementary and Alternative Medicine

Be sure to consider different or "alternative" ideas and approaches to your prescription. If mainstream or conventional western medicine had all the answers, I would not have written this book and you wouldn't be reading it. Complementary and Alternative Medicine (CAM) comprises a field of medicine that includes ideas, treatments and practices such as traditional Chinese medicine, acupuncture, herbs and supplements, prayer and meditation, visualization, and massage to name a few.

Seriously consider everything you learn about. Although much of the field of CAM has not been subjected to rigorous scientific study, that doesn't mean it may not be effective. Even for these treatments and techniques where large medical studies have been negative, a few individual patients may have benefited a great deal but the effect wasn't noticeable in the average of all patients. Perhaps you could be the one to benefit from a treatment that works only for a select few. Don't dismiss the scientific evidence, but review it carefully and make up your own mind.

One word of caution here. There are some truly crazy and harmful ideas out there, especially on the internet. It's okay to be a little skeptical about something that sounds very weird, potentially dangerous or too good to be true. If something smells fishy, discuss it with the people on your team, especially the medical professionals. Use caution here. If you can be sure that it's safe, consider experimenting with it even if it's unusual. If you can't be certain that it's not harmful, leave it alone.

New Ideas for Success

If you want to succeed, *you are going to need to do something different from what you have done in the past*. Of course, this shouldn't be too surprising since what you have done before hasn't worked, at least over the long term. If it had, you wouldn't be reading this book. Many people don't get this and repeatedly "try harder" at the same old plan that has failed in the past. You can believe me (and you really already know) that *trying harder at the same unproductive thing you've tried before is not the answer*. The answer is doing something different.

As we discussed earlier, start by *changing your thinking*. New behavior is called for and that will require new thinking and new ideas—*perhaps even very unusual, or radical ideas*.

Also think about *how* to change, not just *what* to change. Any major lifestyle change is usually hard. How many people do you know that just can't change even though they are facing a grave personal health problem? Bob couldn't.

83

On the other hand, a great deal is known about the process of change, and you need to understand some of it. There are professors who devote their careers to studying how people change. Entire books are written about how to make a change that lasts. This is one of them, but not the only one. Get hold of some others and dig in. You do not want to write another prescription for failure.

And lastly, your prescription will likely need to be out of the ordinary, or "counter-cultural." As we have discussed, to a large extent our thinking and behavior is a product of our culture. What profound force underlies the recent epidemic of obesity and other chronic "lifestyle" diseases? Our genetic makeup, honed by thousands of years of natural selection, did not change in the last twenty years. *However our environment, our culture and our habits have changed big time!*

Simply living in America today has helped to create your current health status. If you want to improve your health, you will need to challenge the usual American way of life — sedentary lifestyle, big portions, instant gratification. *This can be very, very hard.* Most people are pretty concerned about what others think of them. We want to fit in — to be part of the gang. Remember that *fitting in and being part of the gang got you here!* Have the courage to be radically different: to do *whatever it takes* to be healthy regardless of what others think or say about you.

Consider Katie, an Olympic class swimmer who has set extremely high physical goals for herself. In her quest for Olympic gold, Katie has adopted an extreme and counter-cultural lifestyle. Training is essentially a full time job, and she has a personal swim coach to help with that. Equally important are nutrition and rest. Katie maintains a regular bedtime and wake time, sleeping a full nine hours per night. She follows a strict and healthy diet—no junk food, no alcohol and no tobacco - limiting the types of food she keeps in her house to make it easier. Katie follows this regimen seven days a week—no parties on Friday or Saturday night. And she has a regular mental health regimen of meditation twice a day, in addition to assistance from a sports psychologist to manage stress, keep her focused and help her to maintain the right thinking needed to get her to the gold.

You probably don't intend to be an Olympic class athlete, but you see my point. *You can be a gold medalist in your personal health Olympics.* Why be anything less? The champion athlete is not afraid to make a commitment to herself to do *whatever it takes* to achieve victory, and she is not afraid to live in a very different way from most of American society. From a health standpoint, *our culture is toxic. Have the courage to break free of it.*

Be Counter-Cultural

What kind of counter-cultural ideas am I talking about? Let me give you some examples. Watching television is a big part of the American lifestyle today. Many Americans watch twenty or more hours of TV per week. *This is essentially a half-time job.* Multiple studies have shown that on average, the more hours of TV people watch, the more overweight and out of shape they get. This is not surprising, since TV viewing makes it more likely for you to snack and less likely to get physical exercise. In addition, the commercials influence us to purchase more high-calorie unhealthy foods when shopping and dining out.

You may also recognize from your own experience that television can adversely affect your mood. Through intense attention to negative news and ongoing repetition all day every day, news programs very definitely contribute to anxiety and depression in many viewers. More television often equals less happiness. Remember the vast majority of television programs exist for one reason, to make money for the station or producers who are not typically concerned about any adverse effects on your physical, emotional or spiritual health.

Can you limit your screen time? Or can you be more radical and pull the plug? What would happen *if you cancel your cable TV service and go TV free for a month, a year or for life?* How much less would you eat and how much more might you exercise? How much additional time would you have for other higher priority activities? Would you be happier and more optimistic by avoiding the news programs?

Maybe you find that too radical. Okay, what would it be like if you put a treadmill or stationary bike in the living room and only watched TV while walking or biking? How many more calories per day would you burn? How much would your cardiovascular fitness improve?

Does this sound like "crazy talk" to you? Open your mind. Many others have gone TV-free. My family has not had cable or broadcast TV service for over ten years. We miss it a little sometimes but it's been one of the best things we ever did. Some of my friends and co-workers think it's a little strange, but *I need to do what is best for my family and me.* Don't we all? *Don't you?*

It's hard watching your diet and trying to choose foods that are healthy. Reading the nutritional information on the package isn't always helpful either. Serving sizes can be difficult to interpret and even if you understand them, they aren't easy to follow. It's really hard at a restaurant where you cannot be sure of the ingredients, and fat and sugar make everything taste better.

What if you essentially stop eating meals from restaurants or fast food outlets and instead you only eat food that you have prepared at home? You bring a healthy lunch to work every day. Could you do it? Why or why not? How much healthier would you be from that action alone?

What if instead of trying to make healthy choices every time you eat, you simply decided to become a vegetarian or vegan? (Vegetarians don't eat animal flesh but may eat eggs and dairy products. Vegans eat only plant products.) This would make ordering from a menu simpler when dining out and it can be much easier to stick to a healthy diet when you intentionally limit your choices in this way.

Maybe you do pretty well in terms of diet and exercise when you're alone. But, gee whiz, it's really hard to "be good" when you're with your friends. They love to get together after work to eat and drink at the local pub. Some like to smoke, too. You join them with the best of intentions, but after one or two beers, you just can't help getting a burger with fries and a side of onion rings. Afterward, you berate yourself for lack of willpower and vow to "try harder" next time.

Willpower is greatly overrated. Trying harder simply won't work, and berating yourself doesn't help either. How about just not going out with your friends? Perhaps it's more important to control what you eat than to be one of the gang. Or instead, how about suggesting that you go out for coffee as opposed to the burger joint? Can you be honest with your friends about wanting to change and do something better for your health? If not, why not? Do you need to overcome your shyness, or do you need to get new friends?

Get new friends?! Could you really do that? Why not? You know that your friends have a huge influence on you. I'm sure that in your own experience you have known someone who was always a "downer." They were pessimistic and depressing. Whenever you were around them, you always wound up feeling worse. You probably also have had friends who were the opposite, always positive and cheerful, lifting your spirits just from being around. It's important to pay attention to the negative or positive effect that others have on you, and choose to be with those people that help you to be happy and healthy.

You may already know this. Are you a parent? Why do parents care about their children's friends, hoping they'll hang out with good kids and not juvenile delinquents? Because they know how profound this influence is on behavior. Similarly, studies suggest that good health or bad health can be "contagious." People whose friends are overweight tend to get overweight; if their friends get thin then they tend to get thin. If your friends exercise, you are more likely to exercise. If they are couch potatoes, the same can happen to you.

Give this idea real consideration. Your new friends could come from the support groups that we discussed in Chapter 6, perhaps a Weight Watchers group or runners club. Associating with like-minded people is a powerful way to change.

However, knowing is one thing, and doing is another. Right now your friends are either helping you to be healthy or helping you to be unhealthy. *Hang out with the healthy ones.*

Willpower Is Not the Answer

That last example brought up willpower. *I hate the term "willpower!"* Yes, willpower is real and some folks have more of it than others. But no one has enough, and lack of willpower is *not* the problem. The problem is that most people *think* that lack of willpower is the problem. Let me explain.

Let's define willpower as the ability to control your impulses. More willpower is more control, and less willpower is less control. It sounds pretty simple, but your ability to control your impulses is not constant. It varies with the situation. Let's use me as an example. I try not to eat doughnuts, but it can be hard sometimes. Here's a situation from my past as a practicing physician:

It's early in the morning and I've had a good breakfast. On the way to the hospital I pass a doughnut shop, but I don't think about stopping for a doughnut. So far so good. At the hospital where I practice, they have a nice selection of tempting doughnuts in the doctors' lounge/work area. Seeing them, I consider having one but decide against it. This was harder. It turns out that I am scheduled to be on call today and tonight. It proves to be a very busy call day and I am up much of the night with sick patients. I only get three hours of sleep and find myself back in the doctors' lounge at 7:00 A.M. the following morning. I'm tired, hungry, and stressing out over the fact that I have to work until late afternoon before I can go home and rest. My tired eyes catch sight of a tray of delightful fresh doughnuts. You know what happens. I scarf down three of them over the next ten minutes and then feel bad that I did, after which I internally berate myself for a "lack of willpower" and vow to "try harder" next time.

Where was my willpower? I was able to resist the doughnuts when they weren't around. That is, I didn't seek out doughnuts. It was harder, but I managed to resist them when they were present. When I was tired, hungry and stressed and the doughnuts were available, I wasn't able to resist eating three immediately.

You can probably bring to mind many similar situations from your own experience. You may have been thinking that you don't have enough willpower. *Forget willpower! Change the situation.* Alcoholics aren't told to go back to bars with their old buddies and only drink cola. They're advised to stay out of bars and find new non-drinking friends. So too should you concentrate on anticipating your potential weak moments and changing the situation so that you won't need willpower.

Here are some things that I could have done differently:

I could have avoided the doctors' lounge all together. I didn't absolutely need to go there, but it is a convenient place to get organized for the day and I enjoy the company of the other doctors. I could have done the work I needed to do elsewhere in the hospital where doughnuts were nowhere to be found.

Since I knew I would be on call I could have brought a healthy breakfast to work with me the day before. Perhaps low fat cottage cheese and fruit packed in a lunch box. I still would have been tired and stressed, but not hungry when I went into the lounge.

Going forward, I could speak with a few of my doctor friends about this issue. Perhaps many or even most of them are having the same struggle as I am and would like not to be tempted with a doughnut every morning either. We could ask the dietary staff to stop serving doughnuts in the lounge.

Or perhaps I could speak to the one or two close friends that I see almost every morning in the lounge and ask them to help keep me from taking a doughnut. The idea is that when they are with me and I'm about to get a doughnut, they could say something to me like "Pete, you really don't want that doughnut, and you asked us to mention it to you before you eat one."

You can probably think of some additional ways that I might have altered the situation to avoid being tempted by the doughnut that I didn't want to eat. The great secret to controlling your behavior is in *avoiding* temptation, not *resisting* temptation. *Don't rely on willpower. Change the situation.*

Structuring Success

Another way of expressing this concept is the idea of creating structure in your life to leverage your ability to control your behavior. Life used to be more structured than it is now. It was simpler, and there were fewer choices. Most work was physically hard. Even maintaining the home was physically demanding. Foods were less processed and usually healthier. Recreation was physical, not passive as with video games or watching movies on DVD. Today most of us largely have been freed from the need to work hard, and we have more choice in food and recreation. Less structure means more choices of behavior.

You can visualize this concept by thinking of your journey to health and well-being as occurring on a road with many potential wrong turns (Figure 8.1). Wrong turns can represent dietary indiscretions, falling into bad habits or other counterproductive behavior. Taking a wrong turn puts you on the "wrong road" and prevents you from attaining your health goal.

In this model, creating structure can be visualized as straightening the road and eliminating as many potential wrong turns as possible, making it simpler and easier to attain the goal without getting off-track (Figure 8.2).

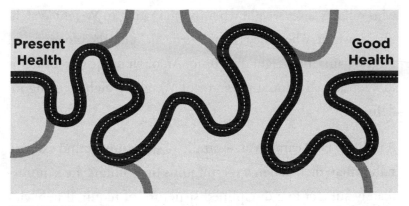

FIGURE 8.1   There can be many wrong turns on your road to good health in our culture and environment.

Imposing structure can be helpful. Most people starting a structured diet, *any structured diet*, will lose weight. It could be the Atkins diet or Weight Watchers or the grapefruit diet. Sticking to the structure or rules produces results. The primary problem is that people eventually stop using the program. I have a friend

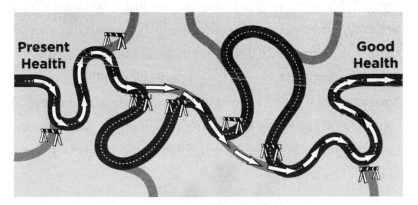

FIGURE 8.2   New structure makes the journey to good health simpler and easier by limiting potential wrong turns.

93

who reliably loses weight when participating in Weight Watchers. However, when she is at her goal, she quits the program and then regains the weight over time. An obvious answer for her is to keep the structured program of Weight Watchers going indefinitely.

A military boot camp is an example of structure around exercise rather than diet. When a recruit joins the military, he is immediately subject to a disciplined structure of required behavior that includes a regimen of vigorous daily exercise. Plenty of food is available, but only at designated times in the mess hall. Initially pudgy, new recruits emerge from boot camp lean and muscled. There was no struggle with willpower or behavior change. The structure assured the desired outcome. Unfortunately these same recruits often regain weight as older non-commissioned officers living in a less structured environment.

I advocate long-term structure, but temporary structure can be very helpful on the road to lasting change too. It takes some time to develop new habits or to completely extinguish old ones. A minimum figure of 21 days is often cited but many habits are more resistant and require a longer period for enduring change. You may find it useful to create temporary structures for several months or more while developing new habits. Once the new habits are firmly in place, the structure may no longer be needed and can be cast off.

For example, Charlie, in attempting to quit cigarette smoking, decides to enforce a rigorous structure of no socializing where he will be exposed to smoking. He completely avoids restaurants and other public places where smoking is permitted. He no longer takes breaks at work with his smoking friends, and doesn't visit his cross-town relatives who smoke. After three months off cigarettes, Charlie is comfortable dining out around smokers, but still feels nervous about hanging out with his still-smoking friends. At six months, he finds that he no longer has any desire to smoke and doesn't require the self-imposed restrictions to his behavior that helped him to finally quit. Way to go Charlie!

Is it possible for you to create structure in your life that helps advance you towards your health goals? Of course it is. A good structure limits your choices so that less or no "willpower" is needed, and healthy behaviors become easier. Canceling our TV service was one way of intentionally creating more structure and less choice in my household. It created more time for learning, conversation and exercise, and less temptation for snacking and sedentary behavior. I am certain that as a family we are less stressed, more relaxed and have a more positive outlook on life from avoiding exposure to the frenetic pace and dire themes of TV news and entertainment.

Intentionally limiting your available choices can be a great strategy for success. Go back and review the examples and identify how this idea of less choice and more structure applies. Give this consideration as you design your program, and try to incorporate helpful structure that you can maintain for the long term.

Take a few minutes and think of what actions you could take to create helpful structure in your life.

Ideas for Helpful Structure (Limiting Choices)

Examples

- ❏ Bring a lunch from home to work every day.
- ❏ Eliminate desserts and junk foods from my home.
- ❏ Restrict TV viewing to 3 favorite shows each week.
- ❏ Exercise before breakfast every day.
- ❏ Only drink no-calorie beverages (water, unsweet-ened tea and coffee, diet soda).
- ❏ Only eat red meat one time per week.
- ❏ Keep fresh fruit for snacking at work at all times.

My ideas

_____.

_____.

_____.

_____.

_____.

_____.

_____.

_____.

_____.

Focus on Where You Want to Go

I have an executive coach at work. She's taught me a lot about changing my thinking. An especially important lesson has been that my mental focus determines the results I get and that subtle shifts in thinking can produce very different outcomes. In business, this means that I get better results focusing on the solutions or desired results rather than on the problems. In clinical medicine, doctors find that patients who focus on being healthy do better than these who focus on the illness. It sounds too simple to possibly make a difference, but seeing a glass as half-full really is better than seeing it as half-empty.

The concept is simply not to focus on the negative or what you don't want. Focus on what you do want. For example, instead of focusing on not being sedentary, focus on being active. Instead of concentrating on not eating unhealthy foods, emphasize eating healthy foods. Instead of fixating on losing weight, dwell on the goal of a lean and healthy body. You get the idea.

How does this work? Focusing on what you want seems to channel your energy in that direction and your brain and body will respond appropriately. Perhaps it relates to our evolution from primitive ancestors. Earlier humans had more primitive brains and I doubt that they were given over to worry about their health or the size of their retirement plans. When they were hungry, they focused on obtaining food. When thirsty they sought water. It seems natural that the mind and body would evolve together to maximize early humans ability to obtain what they were focused on. In any event, it does work. Research it for yourself.

I have a personal, albeit non-medical, example bearing this out. A few years ago I committed to learn to ride a motorcycle, something I had wanted to do for 20 years. In class the instructor taught us to steer simply by "looking where you want to go." Very simply he explained it as: "Look right—go right. Look left—go left. Look down—fall down." From personal experience I can vouch that he was right, when you look down, you fall down. (And it was a brand new motorcycle.) *Focus on where you want to go!*

When you're using willpower, you're focused on the fear of losing control, and you usually end up causing exactly what you don't want to happen. Shift your focus to the positive outcome rather than the fear.

Write the Plan to Win

Once you have gathered together some new ideas, it's time to create your plan. Get another folder or create an additional section in your notebook and write your personal health prescription. Relax, you're not writing a book, just getting down your basic plan on paper. A simple outline or numbered list of items is fine.

Start by clarifying your goal. It's okay if you still have a very general goal such as "to get healthy." However, by this point you've learned a lot about yourself, health and wellness, and any illnesses that you may have. So you are in a good position to firm it up a little. Here are some examples:

- Lose enough weight to stop my diabetes medications.
- Be able to run a mile.

- Be 10 pounds leaner in three months.
- Quit smoking within two months.
- Have enough energy and stamina to play outside with my grandchildren for an hour.
- Complete a 6K "family fun run" and walk event.
- Replace frustration, anger and stress with inner calm over the next year.
- Lose two dress sizes in six months.
- Attain ideal bodyweight, get off all medicines and run a 10-mile race within two years.

Make sure that the target you set is *your* goal, not your spouse's goal for you or something that others think you should do. You decide. And let me repeat that a big commitment to a small goal or general direction is much more powerful than no commitment to an otherwise excellent goal.

Even if the goal is general, it's important that the components of your plan be specific. Remember you're trying to get something accomplished here. For example "eating a healthier diet" is too general to be part of the plan and listing it by itself is not going to be helpful to you. What exactly does that mean? How are you going to measure it? Breaking it down into much more specific components such as "eating two servings of fruit each day" and "limiting bacon to three strips at breakfast one time per week" is much more likely to help you change your habits.

Here are some more examples:

Too general:

- Exercise more.
- Control stress better.
- Be better about taking my prescribed medications.
- Eat healthier foods.

Better:

- Exercise more.
  - Lift weights Monday, Wednesday and Friday.
  - Walk for an hour on Tuesday, Thursday and Saturday.
- Control stress better.
  - Take a class in meditation next month.
  - Join a weekly social group.
- Be better about taking prescribed medications.
  - Put my pills next to my toothbrush.
  - Ask my spouse to remind me every morning to take my pills.
- Eat healthier foods.
  - Replace whole milk with skim milk.
  - Have a salad for lunch three times a week.
  - Only eat dessert on the weekends.

You get the idea. The more specific you can be, the better.

Don't be afraid to rewrite your plan several times before you're satisfied. Use a lot of input from your team and take your time, but don't think it has to be perfect. You can always change the plan when you need to, but remember, nothing happens until you actually start implementing your plan. *A good plan that you actually start is better than a perfect plan that never gets implemented.*

Your team members should help you formulate the plan and should be part of the plan itself. Build into your plan ways they can support you as you begin to implement your program. Perhaps they can call you in the evening and ask how the day went. Knowing that someone is monitoring your progress is a great motivator to stay on track with any program. Perhaps one of your teammates would like to try eating healthy or exercising with you. Or maybe two of you could attend a class on managing emotions together. Keep your team involved and watch great results begin to happen.

Get going. Start now!

Take time to deliberate, but when the time
for action has arrived, stop thinking and go in.
NAPOLEON BONAPARTE

CHAPTER NINE

Follow Up Care: Stay on Track

The doctor's job doesn't end when the prescription is written. She can't just assume that all will go well for the patient and send a big bill. Things happen. Medicines have side effects. Illnesses get worse or fail to respond to therapy. The doctor has to stay involved with the patient and monitor the situation, adjusting the treatment plan as needed for new issues and evolving problems. This is called "following" the patient.

Personally, I've seen many patients with devastating injuries or illnesses who have later recovered from the acute phase of the illness but have severe limitations requiring physical therapy and other specialized rehabilitation. With these kinds of injuries, *the best recovery may be attained only after years of dedicated work by the patient and treatment team.* Usually the road to full recovery is bumpy, with many setbacks and occasional rapid progress. *The people who keep at it and don't quit improve the most.* Perseverance pays off. Hopefully, your journey to health will not be as arduous as this example, but then again it might be. You can get there as long as you are totally committed and *keep at it!*

"Dr. You" should follow "Patient You" very closely. This simply means staying involved by monitoring the plan and how it's working or not working. Don't assume it will work fine from the start, few attempts at major lifestyle change do. So don't give up if it doesn't seem to be working all that well at first. Keep at it. Be a good doctor to yourself and be prepared to adjust to changing circumstances as they arise.

Adjust and Keep At It for Success

Once you've implemented your plan some things will be on track; other things may cause problems. A change in diet might be going great but your exercise regimen is causing very sore muscles or joints. Do you need to stick with it until your body gets used to it? Or are the specific exercises causing a more serious problem? Are your knees really "bad" and running is not good for you, or do you just need new running shoes? Use your team to help you. Hopefully you've included a doctor, chiropractor or personal trainer.

Your problem might be that everything is working great but your work hours change and your exercise schedule is disrupted.

Maybe you are caring for a new baby at home and that affects your exercise schedule, sleep and energy level. Perhaps you built too much willpower into your plan and are finding it hard to resist unhealthy temptations. Get the idea? Be prepared to adjust.

Consider the sailor bound for a new land, who, buffeted by wind and wave on his journey, must take a zigzag course to arrive safely at his destination (Figure 9.1). You too may need many course corrections in your follow up care, adjusting your program to achieve your goal. Review any new issues with your health team. Make the needed changes. *Keep at it!*

Over time, with persistence, you will develop a long-term program that moves you toward your goals. Even then few things work forever. There are countless distance runners who have made running part of their life for decades until a knee injury or arthritis prevent them from running. They then are forced to alter their program to include other forms of exercise. So be

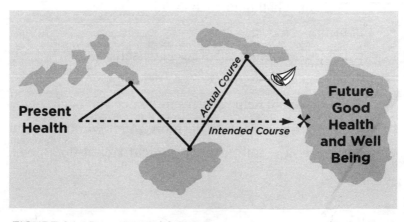

FIGURE 9.1   Be prepared for course corrections on your journey.

comfortable knowing that you too will need to modify your program from time to time. You may need to do it frequently. The key is to *keep doing something that works for you*. If something stops working for you, do something else. *Just keep at it!*

Build On Your Success: Upgrade the Plan

Of course illnesses also get better, and that's where you're going. When an illness improves doctors often decrease the strength of the prescription, *but your prescription is for health*. Be ready to build on your success and take it further. How? Upgrade your plan.

What I'm saying here is that your first plan is just that—a "first" plan. Suppose your initial goal was simply "to be healthier" and your starting plan was very bare bones like this:

- Exercise more.
  - Walk for a half hour each evening.
- Eat healthier foods.
  - Eat fresh fruit instead of sweet desserts.

Will this simple plan help you? Yes, but once you begin to improve you're going to want to do more. After you build your endurance over a month or so you might kick it up a notch like this:

- Exercise more.
  - Walk for forty-five minutes each evening.

- Perform pushups, sit-ups and deep knee bends Monday, Wednesday and Friday mornings upon arising. Work up to 15 pushups, 30 sit-ups and 20 deep knee bends.
- Eat healthier foods.
  - Eat fresh fruit instead of sweet desserts.
  - Reduce red meat servings to three per week.

After two or three months on this program, you would definitely be noticing positive changes in your body and energy level. Here's where you might also upgrade the goal to "lose 10 pounds and get fit enough to play in the company softball league this summer," and decide to try jogging and further changing your diet like this:

- Exercise more.
  - Jog 1 mile Monday, Wednesday and Friday evenings before dinner.
  - Perform pushups, sit-ups and deep knee bends every morning upon arising. Work up to 15 pushups, 30 sit-ups and 20 deep knee bends.
- Eat healthier foods.
  - Eat fresh fruit instead of sweet desserts.
  - Reduce red meat servings to three per week.
  - Drink only no calorie beverages.

And so on. How far can you go? How long will it take? Does it matter right now? Don't limit yourself by seeking answers to these questions too early. Just get started in the right direction and keep upgrading your goals and your plan as your health improves.

My Prescription

Here's how this has all worked for me. My commitment to health began when I was 25 pounds overweight and sedentary. My first plan was pretty basic: to just "lose weight, eat less and exercise more." Obviously, I quickly got more specific, and I did lose the 25 pounds over about six months. I have now committed never to buy a larger size of pants again. I don't weigh myself regularly, but if my pants feel tight, I remember this commitment and immediately take appropriate actions.

Of course, my prescription has changed quite a bit over time, but here's how I would summarize it now: I try to design healthy eating into my life and keep unhealthy foods and eating habits out of my life, so as to not have to rely on willpower. I attempt to ensure that unhealthy foods are not available at home or at work. If they must be present, keeping them out of sight usually helps. I work to never let myself get too hungry between meals and to always keep healthy snacks nearby. I take my lunch to work in order to better control exactly what I'll be eating. Sometimes I do this even when lunch is being served as part of an event I'm attending. I'd rather have control over what I eat.

I've let all my friends know of my preferences and asked them for support. They know that I do not believe in willpower as a way to control my behavior, and that I would rather not be tempted with something bad for me. They know to give me a fruit basket instead of a fruitcake at Christmas.

Through research and trying new things (for example, low fat cottage cheese), I have developed a group of healthy foods that I like and that are good for me. My wife buys a lot of them, I eat a lot of them, and I like it! I don't drink too much alcohol, and take a multivitamin and fish oil supplements.

I exercise five days a week, Monday through Friday, very early in the morning. On weekends I enjoy outdoor recreation, but take a rest from formal training. My workout program has evolved over the years, as I have had to adjust to changing job demands, injuries, illnesses, knee pain, shoulder pain and low back pain. I run twice a week, row (on a rowing machine) once a week and perform resistance exercise twice a week. I keep the workouts short but intense at forty-five minutes or less. To save time in the morning, I changed from working out at the fitness center to exercising in my garage. I go to bed relatively early at night in order to get enough sleep before arising early in the morning to work out.

Just like everyone else, sometimes I have bad days. I may eat candy and junk food, or drink too much wine or skip exercise. Things happen, but so far I've adjusted and I've *kept at it.*

Your prescription won't look like mine, but you may be surprised by where you will take your health as you upgrade your plan little by little. Altering a Chinese proverb, "the journey of a thousand miles is made up of many small steps." *Keep stepping.*

Stay a Student of Health

Even when things are going well, remain enrolled as a student of your physical, mental and spiritual health. Everything that can be learned can be forgotten. Without constant reinforcement, what you've learned could fade away. If you think an article or book is helpful to you, read it again and again until you know it so well that you that it becomes part of your automatic thinking. Do that with this book. If a workout video really motivates you, why not use it frequently?

Also, remember that what you learned last year might not be true this year. Human knowledge changes. That is, things people thought were true last year might not be true in light of new discoveries this year. This kind of change happens constantly in the field of health and medicine. For instance, the minimum recommended daily intake (RDA) levels for vitamins and minerals are changed as more is learned about the positive or negative health effects of these micronutrients. Last year's recommendations may no longer be valid this year.

Another issue is that your learning capacity and receptiveness to new ideas change over time. You may be able to learn something now that you couldn't learn last year. For example, most children are not prepared to learn algebra in the fifth grade, but the same children learn algebra easily in the eighth or ninth grades. This phenomenon isn't limited to children. Many things that I know now and am writing about in this book were not things I learned when I first heard them. I simply wasn't receptive, or they didn't make sense to me *at the time*.

Consequently, you need to keep learning. If you're not learning, your store of knowledge is becoming less and less useful over time. Keep hitting the books, searching the internet, and discussing new ideas with your health team.

You need all the new learning and reinforcement you can get. If you ever think that you've arrived, and you've got everything figured out, you've just taken the first step backwards. Keep the humble "I need to learn" and "I need to change" attitude that got you where you are.

Nothing in the world can take the place of Persistence. Talent will not; nothing is more common than unsuccessful men with talent. Genius will not; unrewarded genius is almost a proverb. Education will not; the world is full of educated derelicts. Persistence and determination alone are omnipotent. The slogan 'Press On' has solved and always will solve the problems of the human race.

CALVIN COOLIDGE

PAUSE FOR REVIEW

Okay. That's it. We're done! Let's put it all together.

1. **Get ready**

   Relying on traditional healthcare is not enough.

   Change your thinking.

   Admit you may be wrong.

2. **Be your own doctor**

   Commit to learning about health for yourself.

   Take responsibility for writing your own prescription.

3. **Be a great patient**

   Accept total responsibility for your own health.

   Be honest with yourself about your health issues.

   Commit to do whatever it takes to improve your health.

4. **Make a diagnosis**

   Identify your problems and their causes.

   Avoid denial.

5. **Assemble your health team**

   Pick people who can really help.

   Build a strong team. Now!

   Include professionals and consider God.

6. **Write your own prescription**

   Do something different, be radical if necessary.

   Customize the prescription to yourself.

   Use your team to find the prescription and to be a part of the prescription.

PAUSE FOR REVIEW

Forget willpower—change the situation.

Focus on what you want.

7. **Follow the patient**

Check on how things are working.

Make changes as needed.

Keep learning and reinforcing your knowledge.

Keep at it!

CHAPTER TEN

Case Study: The Personal Prescription in Action

Bob's Daughter Debbie: A Different Story

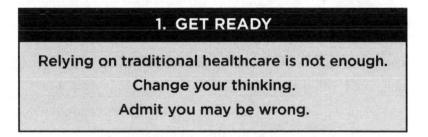

Debbie Baker Williams was 35 years old when her father Bob died of a massive heart attack. She was also a patient of Dr. Lisa Martin for her mild diabetes, borderline high blood pressure, and early osteoporosis.

Debbie was in good physical shape until after the birth of her first child eleven years before, when she gained about 15 pounds that stayed around after the pregnancy. Her second and third child came quickly and, almost before she knew it, she was 45 pounds heavier than when she graduated from high school.

Debbie was a "stay at home mom" who loved being married with kids. Since most of her day was spent tending to the needs of her three children and maintaining the home, she didn't get much vigorous exercise. For relaxation she enjoyed watching television with her husband, Joe, which they did most nights of the week.

She also enjoyed cooking for Joe, who was a real "meat and potatoes" man. Besides generous helpings at meal time, the family enjoyed snack foods and prepackaged desserts. Neither Debbie nor Joe liked alcohol, but they both drank several sodas each day.

Debbie had a tough time watching her father's declining health over the last ten years of his life. In the back of her mind she had a nagging fear of something similar happening to her. Being diagnosed with diabetes had been shocking at the time, but she was taking a pill that was "handling it" and she never could seem to lose the weight or find the time to exercise.

When her father died, Debbie was profoundly affected. During the first few months after his death, she became increasingly concerned and almost obsessive about her own health. She spoke to some of her girlfriends about diabetes and did a little research on the internet which she found alarming. She had never realized just how bad a disease diabetes could be, and she was scared.

---

2. BE YOUR OWN DOCTOR

Commit to learning about health for yourself.

Take responsibility for writing your own prescription.

One day, the little voice in the back of her head that she had been ignoring finally got through. "I've really let myself go. I don't want to go through what Dad did. I have got to do something about my weight. These pills are not the answer." *Debbie was ready.*

---

3. BE A GREAT PATIENT

Accept total responsibility for your own health.

Be honest with yourself about your health issues.

Commit to do "whatever it takes" to improve your health.

Debbie struggled with the idea that she would need to change her life and was depressed that she had "allowed myself to get here." But eventually she decided, "I'm a smart person and I'm going to figure this out for myself. Other people have changed, and I can too! I *am* going to be healthy!"

4. MAKE A DIAGNOSIS

Identify your problems and their causes.
Avoid denial.

Debbie made a list of her formal medical problems—being overweight, diabetes, borderline high blood pressure and early osteoporosis. She added a couple more that she knew were true but weren't really considered significant problems by Dr. Martin—she was generally out-of-shape and had a low energy level.

5. ASSEMBLE YOUR HEALTH TEAM

Pick people that can really help.
Build a strong team. Now!
Include professionals and consider God.

Debbie continued to research these issues on the internet, at the library and with her girlfriends. She knew the basic answer was to get more exercise and take in fewer calories, but how to do it wasn't clear. She made an appointment with Dr. Martin to discuss losing weight and later spent some time with the office nurse and the dietician where she learned a lot. She also prayed about changing, but was too nervous to mention her desire to change to her husband Joe.

She knew that she needed to talk with Joe because it would be hard for her to change if he wasn't supportive. But somehow

Debbie just found it too hard to admit to Joe that she had a problem. Eventually in a quiet moment she broached the subject and immediately broke down in tears. When she managed to get the story out, she discovered to her surprise that Joe was very supportive. It turned out that he had also been thinking that he needed to "get healthy."

6. WRITE YOUR OWN PRESCRIPTION

Do something different, be radical if necessary.

Customize the prescription to yourself.

Use your team to find the prescription and to be a part of the prescription.

Forget willpower—change the situation.

Focus on what you want.

Debbie told Joe that she was developing a plan and wanted to run it by him for input. Over the next week, here is what she came up with:

- Exercise more.
  - Walk for 30 minutes with Kim next door after the kids get on the school bus in the morning.
  - Walk for 30 minutes in the evening with Joe after dinner and before any TV.
- Eat fewer calories and "healthier" food.
  - Eliminate soda and drink water instead.

— Eat more at breakfast and less at dinner.

— Take a multivitamin with breakfast.

Joe agreed it was a good plan and they started that very night after dinner with the walk. Within two weeks they knew that the exercise portion was working—they enjoyed their walks together and didn't miss the TV. But the eating part wasn't going so smoothly—they had a very hard time eating less at dinner and when they did they often snacked on ice cream and other "junk food" later in the evening. Also, they both missed soda a lot, and drank fruit juices "for the taste" instead of water.

7. FOLLOW THE PATIENT

Check on how things are working.
Make changes as needed.
Keep learning and reinforcing your knowledge.
Keep at it!

Debbie went back to the internet, her friends and the dietician to uncover some new ideas. She was surprised to learn that how much food people eat at meals is affected by the size of the plates, the size of the portions and whether or not serving dishes are brought to the table. Who knew that such minor changes could make a big difference? The dietician also startled her by revealing the large number of calories in the fruit juice that she and Joe had been drinking instead of soda. After discussing the situation, Debbie altered her plan as follows:

- Exercise more.
  - Continue the walking regimen as before.
- Eat fewer calories and "healthier" food.
  - Eliminate fruit juice but introduce diet ("no calorie") soda.
  - Keep unsweetened iced tea in the refrigerator.
  - Eat more at breakfast and less at dinner without willpower by:
    - Preparing less food for dinner in the first place.
    - Serving the main dish (usually meat) and any high calorie side dishes (like mashed potatoes) in individual portions from kitchen onto smaller plates.
    - Placing only the salad and vegetable side dishes on the table for family style serving.
  - Eat less junk food without willpower by:
    - Banning junk food and ice cream from the house.
    - Increasing the supply of fruit available for snacking.
  - Take a multivitamin at breakfast as before.

They both started this plan the next day. Debbie threw out all of the ice cream and junk food while the kids were at school and Joe was at work. She made a quick trip to the supermarket to stock up on a variety of fresh fruit. Debbie also started the new dinner plan that evening. Like any change in habits, it was a difficult at first. All three of the children complained about the lack of snack or dessert items, but Debbie and Joe remained patient with the children and committed to long-term change.

Over about six weeks the whole family seemed to get used to the new plan. Dinner went pretty well. Joe was surprised that he was eating a lot less meat and potatoes but was still happy and satisfied with the meals. At first the kids resisted eating all of the vegetables but Debbie and Joe didn't make a big issue of it.

They both still wanted a bedtime snack, but the fruit seemed to satisfy their evening munchies. Debbie was concerned that sometimes the family didn't eat all of the fruit before it spoiled and she didn't like to waste good food. After talking about it with her friend Kim, she decided that it was more important to always have a variety of fresh fruit available than to make sure that none ever spoiled.

At first no one liked the diet soda, but since there were no sugary alternatives, they did drink it. After about three or four weeks they noticed that they actually seemed to like diet soda. They were all surprised at how quickly that happened.

Debbie and Joe did not want to give up ice cream completely, and so Debbie bought a couple of half gallons from time to time. However every time she did, she, Joe, and the kids ate almost all of it within a day or two. After talking about it, they decided as a family that they would not have ice cream at home anymore, but would treat the entire family by going out for ice cream every Saturday night.

As they settled into this new plan over the next four months, things got easier and easier. Both Joe and Debbie began losing their extra weight. Debbie lost about 13 pounds and Joe lost 9 pounds. Debbie was amazed that it didn't seem "that hard" and the whole family looked forward to their Saturday night out at the ice cream parlor.

Debbie and Joe both seemed to have more energy, and felt closer to each other. They were really enjoying their evening walks together and because they enjoyed it so much, they decided to walk a little longer each night. Each was feeling the difference of their change in lifestyle—more energy, more emotional connectedness and better fitness. Not surprisingly, they found themselves making love more often and enjoying it more. They both appreciated that!

Eventually Kim suggested that she and Debbie join the local fitness center with one of her other friends Beth. By this time Debbie *knew* that she *could* make positive changes in her lifestyle, and she had lost her fear of doing something new. She was excited about taking her health and fitness to the next level. They joined the fitness center together.

Debbie, Kim and Beth became workout partners on Monday, Wednesday and Friday mornings. Debbie and Kim continued their walks on Tuesday and Thursday mornings but had gradually changed from just strolling to "power walking." Together with the fitness center staff, Beth who had more experience with fitness, helped Debbie and Kim develop individual strength and aerobic workout programs.

Over the next six months, Debbie was a regular at the fitness center, really working her program. She continued to lose weight, and developed a more shapely and toned body. As she began to see her body change, she felt better and better about her ability to make positive changes and be healthy. She was even more motivated to learn about health and fitness, and began to relook at her diet and meal plan. She became concerned not just about calories and weight loss, but about the actual nutrient and health value of the foods she was preparing for her family.

That brings us up to the present. Debbie has started to prepare meals that are even healthier—lower in calories and higher in nutrients. She has substituted water for the diet soda. Debbie has shed 35 pounds since the beginning of this story. The diabetes and borderline high blood pressure have resolved. She's off the "pills" and, and she feels great. Joe has lost some additional weight just by eating what Debbie prepares along with the nightly walks. He has noticed the changes in Debbie from her more vigorous workouts, and he is considering joining the fitness center himself. The kids still occasionally complain that they don't have cookies and potato chips after school "like everyone else," but Debbie and Joe remain patient with them and explain why "living like everyone else" is not always the best thing to do.

Now, people are starting to ask Debbie how she stays healthy and maintains her weight. *What do you think she'll say?*

Small Start, Big Results

Debbie did it! You can do it too!

Let's talk about Debbie's story for just a few minutes. Although an illustration, Debbie's story is as real as Bob's. Ask your doctor, she's seen this story too. There are many "Debbies" out there. Not so many Debbies as Bobs, but Debbie's story illustrates that *people can and do get healthy quickly once they have made their minds up to do it.* Once you commit to change and then get started, you quickly discover the magic of the "virtuous circle."

You are probably familiar with the concept of the "vicious circle" also called a "vicious cycle." A vicious circle is a chain of events where one negative event leads to other negative events and starts a "downward spiral" of continuous worsening (Figure 10.1).

A health example could be:

Peter regularly maintains his health through a healthy diet and exercise until he develops tendonitis of the right shoulder. He is unable to perform his usual workout for one year because of this chronic problem. After a year of modified and painful workouts, Peter gets frustrated and doesn't exercise at all for the next two months. Also because of the frustration and stress, he eats more

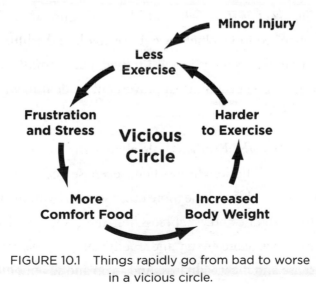

FIGURE 10.1   Things rapidly go from bad to worse in a vicious circle.

"comfort foods" during this time. Pretty quickly he is "out of the habit" of exercise and gains 10 pounds over the next three months. Eventually he decides he needs to get back in the habit with different exercises that he can do. This turns out to be very hard because he's not used to the new exercises, he's out of shape in general, and he is carrying the extra pounds. He feels depressed, exercises only irregularly, and eats more than usual. His weight goes up further, and he gives up exercise totally.

You can see how one bad thing leads rapidly to another in a vicious circle. Slipping into that downward cycle is surprisingly easy to do. It's scary. Be aware of vicious circles and guard against starting down that negative path.

The great news is that wherever you find a vicious circle, you can also experience its opposite, the virtuous circle. In a virtuous circle one positive event leads to more positive events and *things just keep getting better and better* (Figure 10.2). That's what happened to Debbie! Sure it was hard (and a little scary) for her to make changes in her lifestyle, *but she did!* And she stuck with it, and each little improvement made things get easier and easier.

This is how it works! Really! A little change in diet causes a little weight loss. A little weight loss helps exercise get a little easier and more enjoyable. A little more exercise helps with the weight loss. More exercise and weight loss help the energy level and attitude improve. More energy and a better attitude help you with the exercise and the weight loss. And so on and so on. *Things really do just keep getting better and better.*

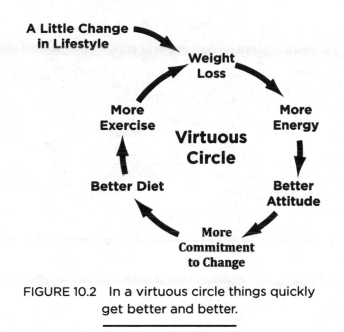

FIGURE 10.2   In a virtuous circle things quickly
get better and better.

Perhaps you have fallen into the downward spiral of worsening health. It's happened to most all of us at some point but *momentum builds in both directions*. One small change can get you started on your virtuous circle back to good health. *Go for it!*

It is not the critic who counts; not the man
who points out how the strong man stumbles,
or where the doer of deeds could have done them
better. The credit belongs to the man who is
actually in the arena, whose face is marred by dust
and sweat and blood, who strives valiantly; who
errs and comes short again and again; because
there is not effort without error and shortcomings;

but who does actually strive to do the deed;

who knows the great enthusiasm, the great

devotion, who spends himself in a worthy cause,

who at the best knows in the end the triumph of

high achievement and who at the worst, if he fails,

at least he fails while daring greatly. So that his

place shall never be with those cold and timid

souls who know neither victory nor defeat.

THEODORE ROOSEVELT

CHAPTER ELEVEN

Total Health:
Body, Mind and Spirit

Throughout this book, I've outlined a framework and general approach for you to use in order to develop your own plan for health and well-being. We have mostly been talking about physical health. In this chapter, we'll move beyond physical health alone to discuss the important interrelationship between your physical, emotional and spiritual health and how it's critically important that each one of these aspects of well-being be improved in order to achieve improvement in the others.

Emotional health is the ability to understand your emotions, remain balanced and deal with life's ups and downs without being derailed. A person who is emotionally healthy is in control of his thoughts and emotions, has good self-esteem and maintains a positive but realistic outlook on life's problems. He might be described as cheerful, calm, even-tempered, and good at getting along with others.

That brings us to spiritual health. By spiritual, I mean issues that concern us beyond our physical form, issues concerning our soul and our very existence. What is the purpose of life? Does God exist? Do I have a soul? Why am I here? How do I relate to everyone and everything else? Does it matter if I live or die? How do I find meaning in my life? How should I live? These are some of the fundamental spiritual questions that we all must face or choose to ignore.

For the purposes of this book, being spiritually healthy means seeking and finding satisfactory answers to these questions for yourself. Spirituality does not necessarily have to involve any particular religion or religion in general, although many people do express their spirituality through one of the world's religions. Now let's see how the physical, spiritual and emotional aspects of life relate to one another and together comprise what I call a person's "total health."

Physical Health: Simple but Not Easy

The "bottom line" for physical health is not all that complicated. All you really need to do is to maintain a healthy bodyweight, eat reasonably nutritious foods, exercise regularly, get adequate sleep, don't smoke, don't drink to excess or use illegal drugs, and don't engage in risky behaviors (for example, driving without seatbelts). Sounds easy, but of course it is not; it takes work to achieve physical health. However, achieving physical health is made even more difficult when the relationship between the physical, emotional and spiritual is not recognized and addressed.

Beyond Physical Health

Too often, mind, body and spirit are treated as separate entities when truly there is only one "you" with mind, body and spirit interlinked, inseparable and interdependent (Figure 11.1).

In my view, each part exists in relationship to the others, and growth or improvement in one area may be dependent upon

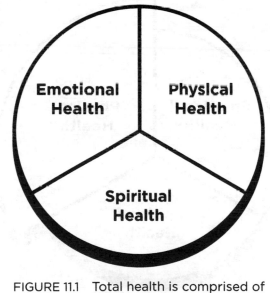

FIGURE 11.1   Total health is comprised of emotional health (mind), physical health (body) and spiritual health (spirit).

the development of the other areas. I'm not alone. According to the American Psychological Association, many Americans say that they have identified this mind-body connection in recent years, and most people now identify stress as a potential source of physical illness. Consequently, It may not be possible to meaningfully improve your physical health without significantly improving your emotional and spiritual health at the same time.

For example, an individual's "total health" may be poor and improvement is indicated in all areas. Yet the individual focuses only on improving the physical, makes some progress, but gets "stuck" because the emotional and spiritual components are now out of balance with the physical (Figure 11.2). Now how,

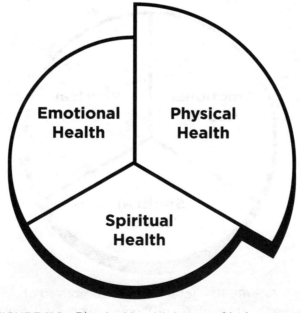

FIGURE 11.2   Physical health is out of balance with emotional and spiritual health.

you ask, can emotions hinder your progress towards physical health? Let's look at this in some detail.

As Thoreau expressed it, "The mass of men lead lives of quiet desperation." How about you? Is your emotional health at its optimum level? Are your emotions balanced to the point that life's ups and downs don't overwhelm you? Here's a simple method to determine the answer:

✔ REALITY CHECK

Do you struggle with any of the following emotions?

- ❏   Depression
- ❏   Anger
- ❏   Hopelessness
- ❏   Irritability
- ❏   Helplessness
- ❏   Sense of Inferiority
- ❏   Sadness
- ❏   Despondence
- ❏   Rage
- ❏   Anxiety
- ❏   Hostility
- ❏   Frustration
- ❏   Resentment
- ❏   Pessimism
- ❏   Worry

Don't be afraid to be honest with yourself and check the boxes. The truth is, lots of people do struggle with these negative emotions.

These negative emotions are common and are therefore "natural" in some sense, but that doesn't mean that they're okay. *They are definitely not okay*, as they interfere with our ability to live in a positive and productive way. These emotions are not only mentally painful; if not addressed they will harm you physically as well.

Think about this for a minute. *Emotions can have direct physical effects*. Stress and anger can lead to high blood pressure, heart attack and stroke. Depression can lead to lower immune function and more frequent infections. Anxiety and worry can lead to sleep loss and chronic fatigue. Here are some classic examples:

- A 54 year-old "Type A, hard charging" male executive dies of an unexpected massive heart attack.
- A 45 year-old woman with depression is "always getting" colds and the flu.
- A 70 year-old otherwise healthy man develops severe depression after his wife dies. He dies unexpectedly six months later of a "broken heart."

Intuitively you know this happens. When you feel bad mentally, you feel worse physically. It works in reverse as well: the physical state can directly affect the mental state.

When you feel good physically, it can lift up your mental health. Perhaps you've had the experience of feeling sad, but after exercising vigorously noticed that you felt better. Exercise is great for directly improving the mood. The exact mechanisms of this effect aren't completely clear, but release of endorphins, which are soothing chemicals produced by the body, may play a part. Regardless, this effect is well documented and important. In fact, therapists may even prescribe exercise as part of the treatment for some individuals battling depression.

Consider these other physical activities or sensations and think about how they might positively affect your emotions.

- Feeling warm sunshine on your skin on the first clear day in spring.
- Making love to your partner.
- Getting a massage.
- Jumping in a cold lake after exercising.
- Relaxing in a hot tub.

What about eating? Can the foods you eat have an effect on your emotions? Of course they can. Why do you think they call some things "comfort food?" Unfortunately, treating an uncomfortable emotional state with eating is just a temporary fix. It doesn't solve the underlying emotional issue and it does create physical problems. Bob developed diabetes and high blood pressure by eating in response to emotional stress, and his stress only got worse in the long run.

Emotions can also have other indirect effects on your physical health by affecting your behavior and your ability to change. Depression, for example, may lead to more sedentary behavior, abuse of alcohol, and changes in food intake with resultant un-healthy weight gain or loss. You can probably understand how pessimism, low self-esteem, hopelessness, and depression could make it difficult to implement the change approach I've out-lined in this book.

Although all components are interdependent, I believe that physical health is most dependent on emotional health, and emotional health is in turn most dependent on spiritual health. Now, I'm not saying that your physical health is completely de-pendent on your emotional and spiritual health, but rather that in order to *fully realize* your optimal physical health, you must have good emotional health, and to *fully realize* your optimal emotional health you must have a secure base of spiritual health.

Given this relationship, you can understand that a frequent pic-ture for individuals who are stuck in their ability to improve their physical health is the combination of: a) physical health limited by emotional health and b) emotional health limited by spiritual health (Figure 11.3).

Here, the emotional health has improved to its limit based on the spiritual health, and the physical health has been limited by a lack of growth in emotional health. Don't get stuck. Grow your total health (Figure 11.4).

I hope that by this point in the book you have seen the value of my approach to physical health and are receptive to more new ideas. The very earliest concepts I covered—accepting that you may be wrong, being open to new ideas, accepting responsibil-

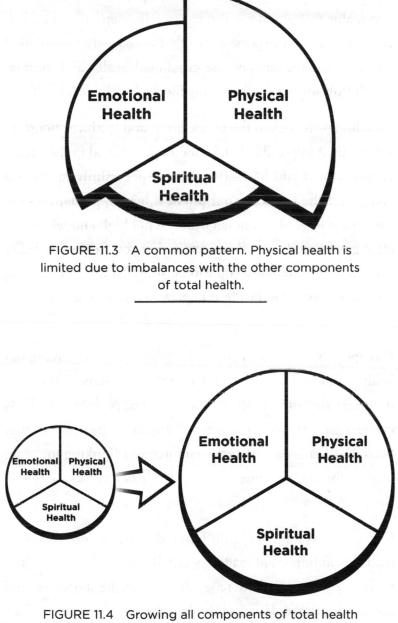

FIGURE 11.3   A common pattern. Physical health is limited due to imbalances with the other components of total health.

FIGURE 11.4   Growing all components of total health in concert is best.

ity, and being honest—are themselves signs of emotional health and maturity. So perhaps you can see how emotional growth could be necessary to physical health. Please keep an open mind and continue reading because emotional health and spiritual health truly are essential building blocks for physical health.

That brings us back to the mind, body, and spirit relationship. If you find it impossible to take the steps outlined in the earlier chapters, or if you have struggled unsuccessfully to make a change for the better in your physical health, perhaps it's because your level of emotional health is not high enough to create a good foundation. If you know that you frequently suffer from negative emotions, you can be sure that they are holding you back. *Emotional health is important and it is largely under your control.*

Perhaps you're saying to yourself, "Wait a minute. Emotional health is under my control? I don't think so." Believe it or not, it's true. Emotions are shaped by thoughts. Negative thoughts create negative emotions; positive thoughts create positive emotions. Furthermore, emotions reinforce our thinking to create more of the same in either a vicious circle or a virtuous circle as we discussed earlier. Here's an example.

Richard's boss was angry with him today over a costly error he made on an important matter. Naturally this bothers him a lot. In the evening, as Richard reflects on his day, he starts worrying about the mistake. He starts thinking that the boss doesn't like his work and that he is likely to be fired. He feels sad and decides to have a cocktail. This makes him feel worse and he begins to ruminate on the consequences of losing his job. Richard starts considering what his family will say, what the neighbors will think and how difficult it will be to find a new employer. "I certainly won't get a good reference. Perhaps I'll even have to move to a new town and accept a lower paying position. This is a disaster." All this time Richard is getting sadder and sadder and focusing more and more on this "very terrible situation." He has a couple of more drinks, wakes up in the morning feeling terrible with a hangover, and gets to work late. As soon as he arrives he's told to see the boss immediately.

What just happened here? Richard entered a vicious circle where the more negative thinking he did about his error and his job, the sadder he became. Going around the circle, these sad emotions produced even more negative thoughts. You can see how his downward spiral originated with his own thoughts. The negative momentum built up fast (Figure 11.5).

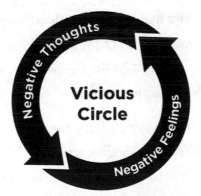

FIGURE 11.5   Negative thoughts and negative feelings form a vicious circle.

However, as we've discussed, wherever you see a vicious circle you can find its opposite, the virtuous circle. You *can* improve your emotions and feel better by directing your thoughts to positive territory.

So how could Richard have handled this situation differently? He could have thought, "Well I did screw up and the boss was angry, but I'm really a good worker and this is my first serious mistake. The boss usually seems to like me. I'm not going to think any more about it tonight, but I'll meet with my boss in the morning to apologize and see where I stand with him. Right now I'm going to clear my head with a good physical workout." If he had been able to control his thoughts in this manner he would not have become depressed.

Now let's get back to the example. Richard has just been asked to see his boss ASAP and of course he is nervous. In fact he's shaky and sweating. Richard just *knows* that he's about to be fired. However, the boss *apologizes to him* for his blowup yesterday! The boss says that although it doesn't excuse his behavior, he has been under a lot of pressure at home and at work. Then he tells Richard that he does great work and that anyone could have made the same mistake.

This illustration demonstrates that emotions don't just happen. They are shaped by your thoughts and then subsequently influence your thinking as we have discussed. Importantly, as the example illustrates, *quite often our thoughts are wrong!* How did Richard's thinking in the example go so far wrong? Basically Richard was assuming that he knew what his boss was thinking.

We all do this way too much, helping to create our own emotional distress.

When you remember that your ability to change your behavior is related to your ability to change your thinking, you can understand why *mastering your emotions* is important to implementing the changes necessary to be physically healthy.

Of course, I'm just scratching the surface of emotional health in this book. Just as with physical health, you will need to do your own learning in this area. I recommend that you research *cognitive behavioral therapy* and *positive psychology*, which speak to this issue. Positive psychology, a new movement in the field of psychology, is concerned with helping people to be happy and experience positive emotions. Cognitive behavioral therapy is very useful in helping people learn to manage their emotions by managing their thoughts. In this type of counseling a therapist helps to challenge the existing thinking that is leading to negative emotions and helps the individual to find new patterns of thought that produce better feelings (Figure 11.6).

Let's go back to our example to see how cognitive behavioral therapy works. If Richard had seen a counselor that evening and shared his thoughts and feelings, the therapist might have asked questions to help him see the potential for errors in his thinking. Questions like these: "How is the usual quality of your work? What does the boss usually tell you about your performance? Do they ordinarily let staff go for mistakes like this at your firm? Can you do anything about it right now?" By reflecting on the answers, Richard might have recognized that he was jumping to

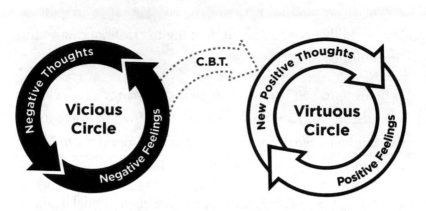

FIGURE 11.6   In Cognitive Behavioral Therapy (CBT), the therapist helps introduce new ways of thinking to the client, helping them to jump from the vicious circle of negative thoughts and emotions to the virtuous circle of positive thoughts and emotions.

conclusions and how he was exaggerating the problem in his mind. Richard could have relaxed and had a good night's sleep.

Cognitive behavioral therapy isn't magic and it isn't "head shrinking." It's simply talking through your thoughts and feelings with someone who can help you see a different point of view. You can see how simple conversation with a caring friend may qualify as therapy. After understanding this and with some practice you can learn to do it to yourself. In my view, cognitive behavioral therapy is one of the greatest health advances of our time. Check it out. *It works.*

Only licensed therapists may diagnose and treat mental and emotional illnesses, but anyone can help you change your thinking. Most of us don't have outright emotional illnesses such as depression or an anxiety disorder. That doesn't mean we never have sad thoughts or some anxiety that may be holding us back; these emotions are "normal" and not necessarily part of a mental illness. But remember, normal doesn't mean good, and not having an emotional illness isn't the same as being emotionally healthy.

Don't be dissuaded if no one you know has heard of this. Many people don't know about positive psychology or cognitive behavioral therapy. Often they are operating on a mental model or worldview wherein harmful emotions, such as depression or anxiety, are believed to result primarily from chemical changes in the brain. This model implies that treating the emotions is best accomplished by fixing the chemical imbalance with drugs. In this example Prozac might be used for depression and Valium for anxiety. Cognitive behavioral therapy operates on a completely different mental model of reality, namely that thoughts cause emotions and that changing your thoughts can change your emotions. In this model, chemical imbalances seen in the brain are *the result, not the cause*, of the negative thoughts.*

Perhaps you're still skeptical. You're thinking, "People don't change their personalities." But you know that they do. Think of an angry young man who becomes a calm and wise old man after a lifetime of experience; or the anxious, depressed drug addict who becomes a wholesome, loving person after rehabilitation; or the hostile, self-centered, greedy businessman who becomes generous and kind after a spiritual experience (think

---

*I'm not saying that all mental illnesses are caused by negative thoughts. Genetics and other biological issues are important causes of mental illness. Medications are a valuable tool in treatment of mental illness, and all treatment of mental illness should be individualized.

Scrooge). The question is, can you change emotionally without a lifetime of experience, without rehab, or without a spiritual experience? Can you change emotionally *now*, just because you want to? *The answer is yes.*

To be honest, I didn't always believe this myself, but as I've shared with you previously I have been wrong about a lot of things. In this case, my mental model was wrong. *Pay attention to your emotional health*. In my experience, most people are a lot more comfortable thinking about and working on their physical health than on their emotional health. Perhaps it's because they are more familiar with the issues involved. Don't worry, you can write a Personal Prescription for emotional health using the same steps we've already covered. Accept responsibility for learning about your emotions and changing them from negative to positive. *You can do it.* As an example, here's my current prescription for my own emotional health.

My Emotional Health Prescription

I try to fill my mind with ideas that help me, often listening to audio books on my commute instead of the radio. I'm also careful to limit my exposure to influences that may harm my emotional development. I don't watch TV and choose my reading material carefully. I select my friends wisely and try not to surround myself with negative people.

In addition, as I mentioned earlier, I have an executive coach (trained as a clinical psychologist) who challenges my thinking, helping me to understand where it may be misguided and negatively affecting me and those around me. My wife and my friends at work are also helpful to me in this regard. I've become willing to talk through my frustrations and fears with them and they help me to see reality. Essentially, they function as lay counselors, administering cognitive behavior therapy as a routine part of my life. I've been considering starting daily meditation for some time but have not yet figured out how to fit it into my schedule.

I'm committed to avoiding denial in any area of my life and actively seek out feedback regarding my performance as an employee, a boss, a husband, a father and friend. This has been hard, as not all the feedback is good, but I've found that the more I admit my mistakes and the more I take responsibility for my own thinking, behavior and emotions, the easier it gets.

Of course I'm not perfect. Sometimes I get frustrated and yell at work, or wallow in depression and self-pity, or get anxious and worry excessively. But then I accept that this is *my* problem and I get back to work on my emotional health. I keep at it.

Your prescription will be different from mine, and like mine, it may not be perfect. That's okay, just get started and keep at it.

Spiritual Health: Often Ignored but Vital

You don't have to grow spiritually if you don't want to, and many people don't. You certainly can be in good physical health and even reasonable emotional health without having great spiritual health or maturity. But don't conclude from this that spiritual health isn't important for your *optimal* physical and emotional health. Good spiritual health provides a better foundation for physical and emotional health.

Think for a minute about people who have experienced extreme tests of their physical or emotional health – prisoners of war tortured for years, concentration camp survivors, bone marrow transplant recipients, war refugees, and survivors of advanced cancer. Great spiritual health is critical in these situations. Many of these individuals attribute their very survival, despite unbelievable physical and emotional stress, to their faith in God or something larger than themselves.

And spiritual health is very closely linked to emotional health. Seeking and finding answers to the big questions of life allows a person to move beyond concern solely for themselves and their immediate circumstances to focus on something larger. In my view, this creates the freedom to grow emotionally.

As we discussed previously, many of the tough emotional issues we face as individuals come from a lack of self-esteem. It's hard not to have anxiety, depression, frustration, or anger if you are constantly concerned with defending a fragile ego, or you have very little sense of self worth. When you are spiritually healthy, you understand that *you matter* and are part of something much larger than yourself.

Speaking only for myself, I believe that God is here, that He loves me and helps me when I ask. I believe my worth as a person comes from that relationship with God, and that I have nothing to prove to others and nothing to fear from others. This allows me to be free to admit my mistakes and errors and to learn from them. With this freedom I am able to change and grow spiritually and emotionally.

I try work on my spiritual health continuously through reading, listening to audio books, prayer, and conversations with close friends. I have two or three breakfast meetings each week with close friends to discuss spiritual issues. Sometimes it's theoretical, but mostly it's practical. How do we deal with life's circumstances, for example, problems at work or at home, within the framework of our spiritual beliefs? Of course we don't always agree, but it helps me stay focused on the big picture. What's life about and how should I live?

But what's right for me won't necessarily be what's right for you. And of course, all your emotional problems don't just disappear because you've grown spiritually. You still need to do the work. Just like being emotionally healthy doesn't make you physically healthy, but it does make it easier to do the work that's required. Spiritual health is the foundation for everything else. Take it seriously.

To summarize, spiritual health nurtures the power to grow emotionally. Positive emotional health allows you to more readily admit mistakes, learn and change. Both spiritual and emotional growth result in positive mental changes, such as increased inner peace, joy and love while reducing anger, worry and frustration. This produces some positive direct physical effects.

Moreover, spiritually and emotionally healthy people are also better able to live a focused, disciplined lifestyle regardless of prevailing cultural norms and values. All of that translates into a greater capacity to take the steps needed to enjoy the rewards of *total health*.

Good for the body is the work of the body,
good for the soul the work of the soul,
and good for either the work of the other.
HENRY DAVID THOREAU

Afterword

Looking Ahead to a Healthier You

Congratulations on arriving at the final chapter in this book! Thank you for reading it. Together we've discussed how the traditional healthcare system may be keeping you from reaching your optimal level of wellness. We've taken a look at the emotions that may be holding you back, and how to turn away from the negatives and embrace better health as something you can achieve. We've worked together to build a team that will support you in your efforts. And we've examined not only how to "tune out" the unhealthy aspects of modern culture but how nurturing your spirit will give you extra strength for the road ahead.

Think about what you've read here and don't just take my word for it. Talk with friends, do some other research, but most of all *try it* and see what happens! I've done my part. The rest is up to you. You *can* be healthy. You *can* take control of your thoughts and habits. But will you?

Yes you will.

You wouldn't have come this far unless you were ready, and being ready is often the hardest part.

Remember what we've covered together. Understand why more medical care won't necessarily make you healthy. Be willing to release old ideas and learn new ones. Accept responsibility for your health and commit to improving it. Ask for help from those who care about you, and assemble your team. Pay attention to your emotional and spiritual health in addition to your physical health. Write your Personal Prescription. Then get started, and adjust your plan as needed going forward. *Jump into that virtuous circle of improving health!*

Believe me, you can do this. Reread this book often for inspiration and to solidify your commitment and understanding of the principles. And please let me know how you're doing with your own Personal Prescription, and any thoughts you may have on this philosophy. My contact information is in my biography at the end of the book.

This isn't rocket science. You know what to do and you don't have to get everything right all at once. If you just start and keep at it, you *will* enter into a virtuous circle. Things *will* get easier and easier. You *will* feel better and better. You may not even be able to imagine how good you will feel as your health improves. In my experience, most people can't. But trust me, *you'll feel great.*

So follow the principles and *keep at it. You can do it! Now, get started!*

The only things worth learning are the things

you learn after you know it all.

HARRY S TRUMAN

Resources

You are going to need to find your own resources, but I thought I would mention some which might help to get started. Here are web sites that I believe to be authoritative and trustworthy sources of health information:

The United States Department of Health and Human Services

- Centers for Disease Control and Prevention
  www.cdc.gov
- National Institutes of Health
  www.nih.gov
- National Institute of Mental Health
  www.nimh.nih.gov
- National Library of Medicine
  www.nlm.nih.gov

- National Center for Complementary and Alternative Medicine
  www.nccam.nih.gov

Major Universities and Medical Centers

- The Cleveland Clinic
  www.clevelandclinic.org
- The Mayo Clinic
  www.mayoclinic.com
- Harvard University's medical school
  www.hms.harvard.edu

Specialty Associations

- The American Academy of Family Physicians
  www.aafp.org
- The American Cancer Society
  www.cancer.org
- The American College of Physicians
  www.acponline.org
- The American Diabetes Association
  www.diabetes.org
- The American Heart Association
  www.americanheart.org
- The American Psychological Association
  www.apahelpcenter.org

Here are some of the books, CDs and DVDs that have helped me along the way. I am grateful to their authors, and it wouldn't be right not to acknowledge them. I hope you find them helpful too, but of course *you* may not. These represent just a small sample of what's out there for you to investigate. Dive in and soon you'll have your own list of helpful resources to recommend to others.

Physical Health

- *Body for Life: 12 Weeks to Mental and Physical Strength* by Bill Phillips and Michael D'Orso
- *Eat, Drink, and Be Healthy: The Harvard Medical School Guide to Healthy Eating* by M.D. Walter C. Willett and P.J. Skerrett
- *Eat More, Weigh Less: Dr. Dean Ornish's Life Choice Program for Losing Weight Safely While Eating Abundantly* by Dean Ornish
- *Pushing Yourself to Power: The Ultimate Guide to Total Body Transformation* by John Peterson
- *Beyond Brawn: The Insider's Encyclopedia on How to Build Muscle and Might* by Stuart McRobert

Emotional and Spiritual Health

- *Your Erroneous Zones* by Wayne W Dyer
- *Choice Theory: A New Psychology of Personal Freedom* by William Glasser

- *Change Your Brain, Change Your Life: The Breakthrough Program for Conquering Anxiety, Depression, Obsessiveness, Anger, and Impulsiveness* by Daniel G. Amen
- *Andy Andrews—The Seven Decisions* by Andy Andrews (DVD)
- *The Traveler's Gift: Seven Decisions That Determine Personal Success* by Andy Andrews
- *The Feeling Good Handbook* by David Burns, MD
- *Living a Life of Inner Peace* by Eckhart Tolle—Audio book (CD)
- *The Power of Now: A Guide to Spiritual Enlightenment* by Eckhart Tolle
- *A New Earth: Awakening to Your Life's Purpose* by Eckhart Tolle
- *The Road Less Traveled (A New Psychology of Love, Traditional Values and Spiritual Growth)* by M. Scott Peck
- *People of the Lie: The Hope for Healing Human Evil* by M. Scott Peck
- *Further Along the Road Less Traveled: The Unending Journey Towards Spiritual Growth* by M. Scott Peck
- *The Road Less Traveled and Beyond: Spiritual Growth in an Age of Anxiety* by M. Scott Peck
- *Authentic Happiness: Using the New Positive Psychology to Realize Your Potential for Lasting Fulfillment* by Martin E. P. Seligman
- *The Spiritual Self: Reflections on Recovery and God* by Abraham J. Twerski

- *How God Changes Your Brain: Breakthrough Findings from a Leading Neuroscientist* by Andrew Newberg and Mark Robert Waldman
- The twelve steps and other teachings of Alcoholics Anonymous (www.aa.org)
- God. You can access him directly through prayer. The Bible may also be helpful. Personally I find that some translations of the Bible can be hard to read and understand, and so I prefer this version—*The Message: The Bible In Contemporary Language* by Eugene H. Peterson

Index

Index

About the Author

Dr. Peter Weiss is a physician, author, speaker and health coach. He has a passion for helping others to become healthier and to learn and grow as people. Of course, he is still learning and growing himself.

Professionally, Dr. Weiss is the former Chief Executive Officer and a member of the Board of Directors of Health First Health Plans, Inc. of Rockledge, Florida. Health First Health Plans is a high-quality, local health plan in east-central Florida serving over 60,000 members.

He attended medical school at Washington University in St. Louis, Missouri. Upon graduation he was commissioned into the United States Navy. He completed an internship at the Naval Hospital, Bethesda, Maryland and then served two years as a General Medical Officer with the United States Marine Corps. Returning to training at the Naval Hospital, San Diego,

California, he completed a residency in internal medicine and a fellowship in infectious disease.

After serving in the Navy, Dr. Weiss entered the private practice of internal medicine and infectious disease in Melbourne, Florida. His success in practice led to an offer to join Health First Health Plans as Medical Director, and he was later appointed CEO.

Dr. Weiss holds Bachelor of Arts and Doctor of Medicine degrees from Washington University in St. Louis. He is a Fellow of the American College of Physicians and a member of the American College of Healthcare Executives, American College of Physician Executives and the American Medical Association. He is board certified in Internal Medicine and Infectious Disease, and holds an unrestricted medical license in the State of Florida.

Dr. Weiss lives in Melbourne, Florida with his wife Sharon. He is an avid gardener and enjoys outdoor activities of all sorts. He also enjoys hearing from readers. Contact him at www.drpeterjweiss.com.